AF870668

# Transgenderism Three

## Transitioning from Health to Infertility

Francis Etheredge

A Biography and Foreword by

Dr. Michelle Cretella

En Route Books and Media, LLC
Saint Louis, MO, USA

ENROUTE
Make the time

En Route Books and Media, LLC
5705 Rhodes Avenue
St. Louis, MO 63109

Contact us at contactus@enroutebooksandmedia.com

Cover Design: Sebastian Mahfood

Copyright © Francis Etheredge

ISBN-13: 979-8-88870-633-6
Library of Congress Control Number:
Available online at https://catalog.loc.gov

All rights reserved. No part of this book may be reproduced, stored in a retrieval system, or transmitted in any form, or by any means, electronic, mechanical, photocopying, or otherwise, without the prior written permission of the publisher or author.

# Table of Contents

# Brief Bio for Michelle A. Cretella, M.D.

**Email:** mcretella@acpeds.org

Michelle A. Cretella, MD, is a pediatrician, researcher, educator, writer, and speaker. She is the past executive director of the American College of Pediatricians (ACPeds) and current Chair of its Adolescent Committee; in this position, she oversees the development of ACPeds' Biological Integrity project. She is a continuing medical educator for the American College of Pediatricians, the Association of American Physicians and Surgeons, the Catholic Medical Association, and the Alliance for Therapeutic Choice. Dr. Cretella is a medical consultant to Alliance Defending Freedom and Liberty Council. She is a peer reviewer for the Journal of American Physicians and Surgeons, Issues in Law and Medicine, and the International Journal of Behavioural and Healthcare Research. She serves on the board of directors of Advocates Protecting Children and the John Paul II Academy for Human Life and the Family. She was a certified Sexual Risk Avoidance educator from 2010 – 2016.

Dr. Cretella served on the Board of Directors of the American College of Pediatricians (ACPeds) for 13 years beginning in 2005, prior to being hired as its first Executive Director, a position she held from 2018-2021. Dr. Cretella served as Vice President of the ACPeds from 2010-2014 and as President from 2014-2018. Before that, she chaired the ACPeds Pediatric Psychosocial Committee, Adolescent Sexuality Committee, and Scientific Policy Committee as a board member. In these roles, she became one of the ACPeds chief researchers, writers, and spokespersons. Her article "Gender

Dysphoria in Children and Suppression of Debate"[1] was published in the 2016 summer issue of the Journal of American Physicians and Surgeons. Through other publications and several media interviews, including a 2017 interview with Tucker Carlson, she became recognized as a leading physician critic of gender ideology. She has contributed to the development and passage of model legislation at the state and federal levels to 1) protect youth from sterilizing sex-rejecting interventions, 2) maintain fairness and safety in female sports, and 3) maintain accurate sex markers on legal documents. She has contributed to several amicus curiae briefs for pro-family and pro-life court cases at the state, federal, and international levels. She has been consulted by Breitbart News, FRC, One News Now, Relevant Radio, FOX News, and many other media outlets over the years.

Dr. Cretella received her medical degree in 1994 from the University of Connecticut School of Medicine. She completed her internship and residency in pediatrics in 1997 through the University of Connecticut School of Medicine at the Connecticut Children's Medical Center in Hartford, Connecticut. She became board certified in pediatrics in 1997 and completed a fellowship in College Health through the University of Virginia in 1999. Dr. Cretella practiced pediatrics with a special interest in behavioral health from 1999 to 2012. She left clinical pediatrics in 2012 to work full time for the American College of Pediatricians and devote more time to her family. Dr. Cretella and her husband are the proud parents of four grown children.

---

[1] https://www.jpands.org/vol21no2/cretella.pdf

# FOREWORD

## MICHELLE CRETELLA, MD

### "Indoctrinating, Diseasing and Sterilizing Youth is NOT Healthcare: Transition and Gender Are Weaponized Words of Mass Destruction"

Author Francis Etheredge uses an engaging, common-sense writing style that helps readers think critically about the claims of gender ideology. This ideology is ubiquitous among children's entertainment, social media, corporations, government institutions, and pre-K through post-graduate education. It is fast replacing Christian anthropology across the Western world, making it a threat to human flourishing. From a medical standpoint, gender ideology and its sex-rejecting interventions, including social transition, puberty blockers, cross-sex hormones, and surgeries, are gaslighting, diseasing, and sterilizing a generation of youth. Contrary to the claims of proponents, they are neither evidence-based nor the international standard of care for youth with gender dysphoria (GD). As a pediatrician and the immediate past executive director of the American College of Pediatricians, I can attest to this.

Since 2019, there have been several high-quality systematic reviews of the world's scientific literature regarding the social, chemical, and surgical reinforcement of gender dysphoria in youth. All have concluded that provision of social, medical and surgical transition interventions for minors is based on low to very low-quality evidence and must be considered experimental. This means the alleged benefits put forth in those studies are likely not true due to significant flaws in the studies' design.[1,2,3,4,5,6,7] As a result, the UK, Sweden,

---

[1]. Department of Health and Human Services, Office of the Secretary. (2025). Treatment for Pediatric Gender Dysphoria: Review of Evidence and Best Practices. Available from https://opa.hhs.gov/sites/default/files/2025-11/gender-dysphoria-report.pdf; accessed April 8, 2026.

[2] Ludvigsson, J.F., Adolfsson, J., Höistad, M., Rydelius, P.-A., Kriström, B. and Landén, M. (2023), A systematic review of hormone treatment for children with gender dysphoria and recommendations for research. Acta Paediatr. Accepted Author Manuscript. https://doi.org/10.1111/apa.16791

[3] Swedish Agency for Health Technology Assessment and Assessment of Social Services' 2019 literature review. https://www.sbu.se/en/publications/sbu-bereder/gender-dysphoria-in-children-and-adolescents-an-inventory-of-the-literature/.

[4] Finland 2020:"Recommendation of the Council for Choices in Health Care in Finland (PALKO/ COHERE Finland). Medical Treatment Methods for Dysphoria Related to Gender Variance In Minors" https://segm.org/ sites/default/files/Finnish_Guidelines_2020_Minors_Unofficial%20Translation.pdf/.

[5] 2020. UK's National Institute for Health and Care Excellence (NICE) reviews:

N.I.C.E. Evidence review: Gonadotrophin releasing hormone analogues for children and adolescents with gender dysphoria.: https://ia802301. us.archive.org/4/items/gov.uscourts.ared.128159/gov.uscourts.ared.128159.
45.9.pdf or https://cass.independent-review.uk/nice-evidence-reviews/; see also N.I.C.E. Evidence review: Gender-affirming hormones for children and adolescents with gender dysphoria.: https://cass.independent-review.uk/nice-evidence-reviews/

[6] Cass Review, Interim Report (2022) https://cass.independent-review.uk/publications/interim-report/

[7] 2022 Florida AHCA Generally Accepted Professional Medical Standards Determination on the Treatment of Gender Dysphoria, comprehensive literature review (Attachment C), Romina Brignardello-Petersen, DDS, MSc, PhD and Wojtek Wiercioch, MSc, PhD: Effects of Gender Affirming Therapies in People with Gender Dysphoria: Evaluation of the Best Available Evidence. 16 May 2022. https://ahca.myflorida.com/letkidsbekids/docs/AHCA_ GAPMS_June_2022_Attachment_C.pdf

Finland, Norway, and Denmark have greatly restricted the use of sex-rejecting interventions among youth with gender dysphoria and instead recommend comprehensive psychotherapy to address underlying issues and comorbid conditions.[8] Most recently, a very large longitudinal registry study from Finland demonstrated that chemical and/or surgical interventions do not improve, and in many cases, worsens subjects' mental health.[9]

### *Gender dysphoria and the harm that follows its social, chemical and surgical reinforcement*

Gender dysphoria (GD) of childhood and adolescence describes a psychological condition in which youth experience emotional distress due to a perceived conflict between their identity and their sex. The associated emotional distress may result in impaired social function. However, when this occurs in the pre-pubertal child, GD resolves in the vast majority of patients by young adulthood.[10] Prior to the 21st century, the international standard of care for GD in children was watchful waiting with or without psychotherapy to identify and treat underlying causes of this disorder. The protocol of socially,

[8] Society for Evidence Based Medicine (2023) "Denmark Joins the List of Countries That Have Sharply Restricted Youth Gender Transitions" Available at https://segm.org/Denmark-sharply-restricts-youth-gender-transitions

[9] S.-M.Ruuska, K.Tuisku, T.Holttinen, and R.Kaltiala, "Psychiatric Morbidity Among Adolescents and Young Adults Who Contacted Specialised Gender Identity Services in Finland in 1996–2019: A Register Study," Acta Paediatrica (2026): 1–9, https://doi.org/10.1111/apa.70533.

[10] American Psychiatric Association, Diagnostic and Statistical Manual of Mental Disorders: DSM-5 (Washington, D.C.: American Psychiatric Publishing, 2013), p. 450-455.

chemically and surgically altering children's bodies to match their irrational beliefs first arose in the Netherlands for only the most resistant cases of pediatric GD. Between 2007 and 2016, however, this "Dutch Protocol" as it was initially called, gradually became widespread across Western nations with social affirmation being recommended for all gender incongruent children regardless of age.[11] The pervasive application of this protocol, *beginning with social transition* for children as young as 18 months of age, and puberty blockers as young as 8 years of age followed by cross-sex hormones, is rooted in the Gnostic myth that a transgender identity is innate. *Significant debate over the pervasive use of this protocol arose because social transition causes persistence of GD which leads to pubertal suppression with gonadotropin releasing hormone (GnRH) agonists (puberty blockers) that are then followed by the use of cross-sex hormones resulting in the permanent sterility of minors as well as other long-term iatrogenic diseases across the lifespan.*

In 2022 the Cass Review Interim Report declared "it is important to view [social transition] as an active intervention because it may have significant effects on the child or young person in terms of their psychological functioning" (p.62).[12] Social transition refers to active behavioral interventions undertaken by family, peers and community members reinforcing a child's discordant identity. These active interventions include endorsing a change in name, pronoun use, hair

---

[11] Rafferty J. Ensuring Comprehensive Care and Support for Transgender and Gender-Diverse Children and Adolescents. Pediatrics (2018). Available at https://publications.aap.org/pediatrics/article/142/4/e20182162/37381/Ensuring-Comprehensive-Care-and-Support-for?autologincheck=redirected

[12] Cass Review, Interim Report (2022) https://cass.independent-review.uk/publications/interim-report/

style, and clothing that match the child's discordant identity, and allowing the child access to spaces and activities normally reserved for the opposite sex. Some claim that families who affirm their children's gender dysphoria or trans-identities improve their children's mental health citing studies by Olson, et al. (2016) and Durwood, McLaughlin and Olson (2017).[13,14] However, this claim was proven false once statistical errors were corrected.[15] The original studies were reassessed by Schumm and Crawford in 2019 who reported, "[A] reanalysis of their findings [reveals] slightly higher levels of depression but significantly and substantively meaningful differences in anxiety and self-worth, and with results favoring cisgender children, even when the transgender children had high levels of parental support for their gender transitioning." [31] Therefore, affirming social transition in and by families does not benefit gender dysphoric /trans-identified children.

Similar negative conclusions have been drawn regarding social transition more broadly. In April 2022, Hall and colleagues published a systematic review and narrative summary of the literature on social transitioning for children and adolescents. They found that the 10 studies that qualified for inclusion were generally "of low

---

[13] Olson, Kristina R., Lily Durwood, Madeleine DeMeules, and Katie A. McLaughlin. 2016b. "Mental Health of Transgender Children Who Are Supported in Their Identities." Pediatrics 137:e20153223.

[14] Durwood, Lily, Katie A. McLaughlin, and Kristina R. Olson. 2017. "Mental Health and Self-worth in Socially Transitioned Transgender Youth." Journal of the American Academy of Child & Adolescent Psychiatry 57:116–23.

[15] Schumm, Walter & Crawford, Duane. (2019). Is Research on Transgender Children What It Seems? Comments on Recent Research on Transgender Children with High Levels of Parental Support. The Linacre Quarterly. 87. 002436391988479. 10.1177/0024363919884799.

quality," because they were mostly from the United States, and used community samples and cross-sectional analyses. There were no high quality prospective longitudinal studies with appropriate comparator groups assessing the impact of social transition on mental health or gender-related outcomes in children or adolescents. Hall and colleagues concluded, "Overall studies consistently reported no difference in mental health outcomes for children who socially transitioned across all comparators. Studies found mixed evidence for adolescents who socially transitioned." Stated differently, this systematic and narrative review of the best studies on social transition found no evidence social transition reduces suicidality or confers any mental health benefit to gender dysphoric youth.[16] The final Cass Review published in 2024 reached the same conclusion.[17]

In contrast to social transition, the quality of family and peer relationships does correlate with gender dysphoric children's mental health. A 2021 study from the Hamburg Gender Identity Service entitled, "Not social transition status, but peer relations and family functioning predict psychological functioning in a German clinical sample of children with gender dysphoria" bluntly declares, "Therefore, claims that gender affirmation through transitioning socially is beneficial for children with [gender dysphoria or trans-identities] could not be supported from the present results. Instead, the study highlights the importance of individual social support provided by

---

[16] Hall R, Taylor J, Hewitt CE, *et al*, Impact of social transition in relation to gender for children and adolescents: a systematic review. *Archives of Disease in Childhood* Published Online First: 09 April 2024. doi: 10.1136/archdischild-2023-326112

[17] Cass Review (2024) https://cass.independent-review.uk/wp-content/uploads/2024/04/CassReview_Final.pdf

peers and family, independent of exploring additional possibilities of gender transition during counseling."[18]

***Social transition prevents desistance and can lead to irreversible medical damage***

As previously stated, the natural course of gender dysphoria is desistance by adulthood, conservatively in 85 percent, unless it is affirmed.[19] However, social transition leads to persistence of gender dysphoria. The pro-transition Endocrine Society guidelines state, "Social transition is associated with the persistence of [gender

---

[18] Sievert ED, Schweizer K, Barkmann C, Fahrenkrug S, Becker-Hebly I. Not social transition status, but peer relations and family functioning predict psychological functioning in a German clinical sample of children with Gender Dysphoria. Clin Child Psychol Psychiatry. 2021 Jan;26(1):79-95. doi: 10.1177/1359104520964530. Epub 2020 Oct 20. PMID: 33081539.

[19] American Psychiatric Association. (2013). Diagnostic and statistical manual of mental disorders (5th ed.). Arlington, VA: American Psychiatric Publishing. P.455; See also Bockting, W. (2014). Chapter 24: Transgender Identity Development. In Tolman, D., & Diamond, L., Co-Editors-in-Chief (2014) *APA Handbook of Sexuality and Psychology* (2 volumes). Washington D.C.: American Psychological Association, *1*: 744.); See also Singh D, Bradley SJ and Zucker KJ (2021) A Follow-Up Study of Boys With Gender Identity Disorder. *Front. Psychiatry* 12:632784. doi: 10.3389/fpsyt.2021.632784; See also Hembree, W., Cohen-Kettenis, et al., (2017) Endocrine treatment of gender-dysphoric/gender-incongruent persons: An Endocrine Society clinical practice guildeline. J Clin Endocrinol Metab,102:1–35.; See also Zucker, K. J. (2018). The myth of persistence: response to "A critical commentary on follow-up studies and 'desistance' theories about transgender and gender nonconforming children" by Temple Newhook et al. International Journal of Transgenderism, 19(2), 231–245. Published online May 29, 2018. http://doi.org/10.1080/15532739.2018.1468293

dysphoria] as a child progresses into adolescence."[20] Psychologist Ken Zucker found, "Gender social transition of prepubertal children will increase dramatically the rate of gender dysphoria persistence," and that it "might be characterized as iatrogenic."[21] In other words, social transition interferes with the natural desistance of gender dysphoria sending more youth onto the medical and surgical transition pathway. The 2024 Final Cass Review paragraph 76 noted, "The systematic review showed no clear evidence that social transition in childhood has any positive or negative mental health outcomes, and relatively weak evidence for any effect in adolescence. ***However, those who had socially transitioned at an earlier age and/or prior to being seen in clinic were more likely to proceed to a medical pathway*** (emphasis mine)."[34]

Puberty is not a disease. It is a critical window of normal physical, cognitive, emotional, psychological, social and spiritual development that is masked by social transition and permanently disrupted by puberty blockers. When normal puberty is socially masked and artificially arrested with puberty blockers, valuable time is forever stolen from these children, time that should be spent in normal development. This time, during which highly significant and irreplaceable advances in bone, brain, social, emotional, spiritual and sexual maturation occur, is time in normal and active psychosocial and physical development – that can never be given back.

---

[20] Hembree, W., Cohen-Kettenis, et al., (2017) Endocrine treatment of gender-dysphoric/gender-incongruent persons: An Endocrine Society clinical practice guildeline. J Clin Endocrinol Metab,102:1–35.

[21] Zucker, K.J. (2020), Debate: Different strokes for different folks. Child Adolesc Ment Health, 25: 36-37. https://doi.org/10.1111/camh.12330

Puberty blockers arrest pubertal development by acting on the brain. Boys are chemically castrated and girls are chemically driven into premature menopause for as long as the puberty blockers are used. This developmental arrest can result in permanent sexual dysfunction, infertility, bone loss, and potentially altered brain development with cognitive impairment.[22,23] When gender-dysphoric youth are socially transitioned and given puberty blockers nearly 100% of them go on to identify as 'transgender' and request cross-sex hormones.[24] *This suggests that social transition and puberty blockers*

---

[22] Laidlaw M, Van Meter QL, Hruz PW, Van Mol A and Malone WJ. *The Journal of Clinical Endocrinology & Metabolism*, 2019;104(3): 686–687, https://doi.org/10.1210/jc.2018-01925

[23] Vigil P, et al., "Endocrine Modulation of the Adolescent Brain: A Review" *Journal of Pediatric & Adolescent Gynecology* 24(6):330-337 (December 2011). See also Craig MC, Fletcher PC, Daly EM, Rymer J, et al. Gonadotropin hormone releasing hormone agonists alter prefrontal function during verbal encoding in young women. Psychoneuroendocrinology. 2007;32(8-10):1116-27. DOI:10.1016/j.psyneuen.2007.09.009; Christian J. Nelson, et al., "Cognitive Effects of Hormone Therapy in Men With Prostate Cancer" *Cancer* 113(5):1097-1106 (2008).

[24] Brik T, Vrouenraets LJJJ, de Vries MC, Hannema SE. Trajectories of adolescents treated with gonadotropinreleasing hormone analogues for gender dysphoria [published online ahead of print March 9, 2020]. Arch Sex Behav. doi:10.1007/s10508-020-01660-8; Kuper LE, Stewart S, Preston S, Lau M, Lopez X. Body dissatisfaction and mental health outcomes of youth on gender-affirming hormone therapy. Pediatrics. 2020;145(4):e20193006; Annelou L.C. de Vries, et al., "Puberty suppression in adolescents with gender identity disorder: A prospective follow-up study" *The Journal of Sexual Medicine* 8(8): 2276–2283 (2011). Wiepjes CM, Nota NM, de Blok CJM, et al. The Amsterdam cohort of gender dysphoria study (1972-2015): trends in prevalence, treatment, and regrets. J Sex Med. 2018;15(4):582–590; Carmichael P, Butler G, et al. Short-term outcomes of pubertal suppression in a selected cohort of 12 to 15 year old young people with

*"lock" kids into their gender confusion.* As a result, these children who have their development blocked in early puberty, and are later given cross-sex hormones, will be permanently sterilized rather than healed.[26,25] Cross-sex hormones also put these youth at an increased risk of heart attacks, stroke, diabetes, blood clots, cancer and other diseases across their lifespan.[26,26]

### *Social and medical transition do not prevent suicide*

Nevertheless, some transgender affirming ideologues insist these harms must be accepted because social affirmation, blockers, hormones and surgeries prevent youth suicide. This too is false. In reality, suicide risk among trans-identifying youth is similar to the elevated suicide rates among other at-risk youth. Based upon data from the United Kingdom's Tavistock Gender Identity Clinic, Oxford sociologist, Dr. Michael Biggs, has reported that being trans-identified increases suicide risk by a factor of 13. He notes that this

---

persistent gender dysphoria in the UK. medRxiv 2020.12.01.20241653.

[25] Leena Nahata, et al., "Understudied and Under-Reported: Fertility Issues in Transgender Youth—A Narrative Review" *Journal of Pediatrics* 205:265-271 (February 2019)

[26] Dorte Glintborg, Katrine Hass Rubin, Tanja Gram Petersen, Øjvind Lidegaard, Guy T'Sjoen, Malene Hilden, Marianne Skovsager Andersen, Cardiovascular risk in Danish transgender persons: a matched historical cohort study, *European Journal of Endocrinology*, Volume 187, Issue 3, Sep 2022, Pages 463–477, https://doi.org/10.1530/EJE-22-0306; Talal Alzahrani, et al., "Cardiovascular Disease Risk Factors and Myocardial Infarction in the Transgender Population" *Circulation* 12(4):e005597 (2019); Katrien Wierckx, et al., "Prevalence of cardiovascular disease and cancer during cross-sex hormone therapy in a large cohort of trans persons: a case-control study" *European Journal of Endocrinology* 169(4):471-478 (2013).

elevated risk, while concerning, is less than or within range of the suicide risk associated with other disorders: anorexia increases suicide risk by a factor of 18; depression multiplies one's risk by a factor of 20, and autism raises suicide risk by a factor of 8. Anorexia, depression and autism also often coincide with gender dysphoria.[27] Although individuals may report a "honeymoon period" of relief and happiness with the cosmetic results from cross-sex drugs and surgeries, these interventions do not improve mental health in the long-term. A thirty year study of a large population of transgender-identified adults who used hormones and surgeries to impersonate the opposite sex (in LGBT-affirming Sweden) found that their mental health was significantly worse than that of the general population ten years after surgery and by the conclusion of the study, their completed suicide rate was 19 times greater than that of the general population.[28] A very large longitudinal registry study from Finland (2026) demonstrated that sex-rejecting medical and surgical procedures correlate with a significant worsening of mental health for gender distressed youth.[29] *In short, suicide prevention for youth with gender dysphoria should be the same as it is for all other at risk youth;*

---

[27] Biggs M. Suicide by trans-identified children in England and Wales (October 2018). Available at: https://www.transgendertrend.com/suicide-by-trans-identified-children-in-england-and-wales/

[28] Cecilia Dhejne, et al., "Long-Term Follow-Up of Transsexual Persons Undergoing Sex Reassignment Surgery: Cohort Study in Sweden" *PLOS One* 6(2):e16885 (2011) available at https://journals.plos.org/plosone/article?id=10.1371/journal.pone.0016885

[29] S.-M.Ruuska, K.Tuisku, T.Holttinen, and R.Kaltiala, "Psychiatric Morbidity Among Adolescents and Young Adults Who Contacted Specialised Gender Identity Services in Finland in 1996–2019: A Register Study," Acta Paediatrica (2026): 1–9, https://doi.org/10.1111/apa.70533.

*namely, individual and family counseling to identify and resolve underlying issues, and psychiatric medications when indicated.*

### Concluding remarks

In the following chapters, Etheredge first illustrates that few things on the road to adult identity are permanent. Next, he allows his readers to reason through the many logical results of gender ideology's deceitful language. Finally, he asks if the professional "fence sitters" who posit that there may be some youth who would benefit from destructive sex-rejecting procedures are correct – that rigorous randomized clinical trials of sex-rejecting interventions are required.

Ultimately, an ethical society promotes policies that maximize and/or restore normal development, health and function, and relieve suffering. The majority of youth with gender dysphoria are recognized to suffer from preceding unresolved traumas, neurodiversity and/or mental disorders. The use of social reinforcement, puberty blockers, cross-sex hormones and cross-sex surgeries, do not mitigate or heal these underlying issues, nor do they improve mental health or prevent suicide in the long term. *Instead, sex-rejecting interventions disrupt normal mental and physical health, function and development. In fact, social reinforcement of the sex-rejecting "transgender" ideology leads to medical and surgical interventions that can permanently sterilize, disease and mutilate these emotionally distressed youth.* This seems to me a modern form of eugenics. See if you agree.

## INTRODUCTION

# WHAT IS "TRANSITIONING"?

> 'St. Teresa Benedicta of the Cross says to us all: *Do not accept anything as the truth if it lacks love. And do not accept anything as love which lacks truth!* One without the other becomes a destructive lie' (6) 1

On the one hand, an individual has sued those responsible for the fact that, at '16, Fox underwent a double mastectomy to remove her [healthy] breasts. Very soon after, she regretted the life-altering surgery'; and, in addition, other lawsuits are pending.[2] On the other hand, The Federal Trade Commission (FTC) of America is suing the World Professional Association for Transgender Health (WPATH).[3] And, as we shall see in the course of this book, and particularly towards the end of it, there is no need for a proposed puberty blocker experiment on 11–12-year-olds in the UK[4]; the evidence is already in that transitioning is harmful and, if it has been medicalized, often

---

[1] Homily of John Paul II for the Canonization of Edith Stein, Sunday, 11 October, 1998.

[2] Brian Chai, February 13th, 2026, "Detransitioner Fox Varian Awarded $2 Million in Historic Lawsuit: A young woman who had her healthy breasts removed at age 16 was awarded millions after she filed a malpractice lawsuit against the doctors who pushed her towards "gender transition": https://adflegal.org/article/detransitioner-fox-varian-awarded-2-million-in-historic-lawsuit/.

[3] This is discussed more fully at the end of this book, "Postscript: Evidence or a Smoke Screen?"

[4] "Appendix: Do we need another puberty-blocker trial?"

irreversible. Indeed, because of recent comments by WPATH, saying that their guidelines are 'opinions' in an 'area of significant medical debate', there are a number of people calling for a review of any guidelines based on what has hitherto been published.[5] Note, too, that America is now challenging the 2019 'reclassification [of 'gender dysphoria' as a medical condition by the World Health Organization, so that it can be treated] through pharmacological and surgical interventions [as] a matter of course instead of mental health and psychosocial support, as before.' The American intervention is seeking to reassert the need for 'governments to explore alternatives to sex-rejecting procedures and to ensure that children who experience gender dysphoria have access to mental health and psychosocial support.'[6] Thus, in keeping with what is possibly going to be a review of WPATH's guidelines across the world, it would be more than advisable for any organization, including the UK puberty-blocker trial, to abandon its proposed experiment on 11–12-year-olds.

### *The possibility of the fraudulent use of endocrine codes*

To continue, WPATH is the international body that claims to be a specialist in transgender care, 'founded in 1979'. WPATH is being sued for false claims by the Federal Trade Commission; and, as such,

---

[5] Rachel Baxendale, August 15th, 2026, "Pressure mounts on Butler to review gender care after WPATH admission: The world's leading transgender health authority has told a US court its treatment guidelines are 'opinions' – raising serious questions over care of Australian children": https://archive.md/C1LCY#selection-773.0-777.170.

[6] Stefano Gennarini, 2026, "U.S. Takes on Global Trans at the UN": https://c-fam.org/friday_fax/us-takes-on-global-trans-at-the-un/.

it is said to hide risks, exaggerate benefits, claiming that medical procedures were necessary – even if WPATH claims that the applicability of their advice has to be determined on an individual-by-individual basis[7]. WPATH, in its submission, denies that it is not responsible for how its advice is actioned; and, in general, distances itself from what is done by those actioning treatments for young people who suffer a discrepancy, as it were, between their sex from conception and how they feel about it in the course of growing up. On the other hand, if WPATH training materials advocate the use of clinically inappropriate codes for prescribing and charging for puberty blockers, then this seems to establish a link between WPATH and fraud: 'Begin[ing] with a 2021 training presentation by two physicians, entitled "Insurance Coverage and Coding Considerations." This presentation is best read as promoting the misleading use of several ICD-10 codes.' [8] There is now widespread evidence of the misuse of

---

[7] Calvin Freiburger, June 18th, 2026, "Trump admin sues top pro-LGBT medical group over 'false' claims on child 'transitions': Federal regulators and four states accuse WPATH of hiding risks, exaggerating benefits, and falsely portraying pediatric 'gender transition' procedures as 'medically necessary'"; references to WPATH's individualised approach are on pp. 5, 18, 23-24: https://www.lifesitenews.com/news/trump-admin-sues-top-pro-lgbt-medical-group-over-false-claims-on-child-transitions/?utm_source=digest-2026-06-18&utm_medium=email; and in the following, standard WPATH guidance, there are many references to this emphasis on the individualised assessment of each person, eg. Pp. 46, 54, 56-57, 59, 65, 67, 69 etc. as found in E. Coleman, A. E. Radix, W. P. Bouman, et al. (2022) Standards of Care for the Health of Transgender and Gender Diverse People, Version 8, International Journal of Transgender Health, 23:sup1, S1-S259, DOI: https://www.tandfonline.com/doi/pdf/10.1080/26895269.2022.2100644.

[8] P. 20 of "Wolves in White Coates: How Doctors and Hospitals Pushed and Profited from the Fraud of "Gender Medicine"", 2026, Make America Healthy Again: https://www.hhs.gov/sites/default/files/hhs-wolves-in-white-coats.pdf.

endocrine codes, particularly one where it is stated to be 'unspecified', in order to obtain money to pay the prescription fee for hormones for young people: 'The report [Wolves in White Coats] also analyses nationwide claims data from 2015 through 2025 and identifies approximately $50 million in insurance claims for puberty blockers billed using endocrine disorder diagnostic code E34.9 (Endocrine Disorder, Unspecified)'.[9] The doses of these hormones, as discussed in a previous work, are often not only unnecessary but are exceedingly high and damaging[10].

### *Compromised objectivity: WPATH membership and that of other organizations*

Note, too, the overlap between membership of WPATH and the policies advocated by the Endocrine Society in 2017, the American Psychological Association in 2015, and the American Academy of Pediatrics in 2016, all advocating pro-transgender medicalization

---

[9] August 13th, 2026, "HHS Releases Report Exposing Fraudulent Insurance Coding For Sex-rejecting Procedures On Minors": https://www.hhs.gov/ pressroom/hhs-report-insurance-coding-sex-rejecting-procedures-minors.html.

[10] Etheredge, *Transgenderism Two: Evidence and Identity*; cf. also the ITEST [Institute for Theological Encounter with Science and Technology] webinar, *Scientific, Clinical, & Theological Problems with the Gender Dysphoria Affirmation Model* with presenters Stephen Rouhana, Ph.D. and Paul Hruz, M.D., Ph.D [endocrinologist]": https://www.youtube.com/watch?v= zg8Fp0X2kyw. And Stephen gives a good background account of how the changing classifications of gender dysphoria led to enabling insurance claims to be for the medicalized 'gender-affirming-care' e.g. drugs, surgeries etc.

practices[11]. In Australia, there appears to be a conflict of interest, for the following reason: ‘The Australian Health Practitioner Regulation Agency [AHPRA] surfaced a six-month-old anonymous complaint against Professor Gary Geelhoed within days of him challenging AHPRA over its treatment of Queensland psychiatrist Dr Andrew Amos’ who also objects to gender-affirming-care’s ‘medical treatments’[12]. Moreover, Professor Geelhoed questioned “‘AHPRA’s close association with (trans activist) organisations such as ACON’; and, therefore, AHPRA’s ‘impartiality when adjudicating what are fundamentally clinical and scientific matters’”. Geelhoed has stridently and forcefully objected to the ‘mutilation’ of children by so called ‘gender-affirming-care’[13]. See, also, another conflict of interest: the compromising of the impartiality of police and the public right to be stopped and searched by a man or a woman who is actually the same sex as the person stopped. Thus, some of the UK police who are said to be ‘gender-fluid’ are being issued with “dual” identities as “male” or “female” when it comes to being able to do ‘stop and search’

---

[11] Pages 42-43 of “Wolves in White Coates: How Doctors and Hospitals Pushed and Profited from the Fraud of “Gender Medicine””, 2026.

[12] Stephen Rice, April 24th, 2026, “‘Take my treatment as a warning’: Psychiatrist suspended for opposing youth gender treatments: Psychiatrists pleaded with professional body to support outspoken colleague Andrew Amos, only to discover it had suspended him”: https://archive.md/2dtEi.

[13] Bernard Lane, August 19th, 2026, “Top pediatrician faces probe after questioning health regulator’s impartiality: A distinguished pediatrician who publicly condemned transgender mastectomies for minors has been hit with a complaint by AHPRA, days after challenging the regulator”: https://archive.md/1zBgS.

activities: Some forces 'had issued more than one card to officers who said they identified as both male and female.'[14]

Thus, the question arises and remains, is this "distancing" justified when WPATH has claimed almost privileged competence in the field of gender-affirming-care? This lawsuit, between the FTC in America and WPATH, is also in the context of recent reports questioning the validity of 'gender affirming care'[15]. Indeed, while WPATH's submission acknowledges the existence of reports that challenge their claims[16], there is a disregard for the fact that the

---

[14] Hayley Dixon, 23rd August, 2026, "Gender-fluid police given male and female warrant cards:

Officers who identify as both men and women issued with two sets of identity documents": https://archive.ph/e9Q1q#selection-2135.4-2139.90.

[15] Cf. Etheredge, *Transgenderism: A Question of Identity*, discusses the Cass Report; and cf. Etheredge, *Transgender Two: Evidence and Identity*, which includes a discussion on the American report on Paediatric Health with particular reference to gender affirming care. Both books draw on innumerable other sources too.

[16] UNITED STATES DISTRICT COURT FOR THE NORTHERN DISTRICT OF TEXAS FORT WORTH DIVISION. FEDERAL TRADE COMMISSION, et al., Plaintiffs, v. WORLD PROFESSIONAL ASSOCIATION FOR TRANS-GENDER HEALTH, INC., a Texas corporation, et al., Defendants. Case No. 4:26-cv-00748-O

DEFENDANT WORLD PROFESSIONAL ASSOCIATION FOR TRANSGENDER HEALTH, INC.'S MEMORANDUM IN SUPPORT OF ITS MOTION TO DISMIS, p. 1: https://segm.org/sites/default/files/2026-08/WPATH%20Motion%20to%20dismiss_Aug%202026.pdf. Cf. Pp. 6, 33 that reference the Cass Report; and cf. P. 35 of WPATH's submission, which says: 'As Plaintiffs allege, in "November 2025, the U.S. Department of Health and Human Services published a 400-page report titled 'Treatment for Pediatric Gender Dysphoria: Review of Evidence and Best Practices' ('The HHS Report'), which assessed the evidence base for the medical interventions on children that WPATH recommends and concluded that it is exceptionally weak." Compl. ¶ 25. The federal government has thus already alerted doctors and the public to what it views as the problems with WPATH's speech. That is the exact remedy the First Amendment envisions: "the surgical removal of healthy body parts is, in effect, a wound with lasting implications for the person upon whom this action was carried out. The technical word for harm caused by some kind of medical intervention is iatrogenic: 'Iatrogenesis [or iatrogenic harm] may thus include mental suffering via medical beliefs or a practitioner's statements.'[17] Thus, in the field of gender affirming care, there is a wide scope for claimants arguing that they have suffered not only physical harm but 'mental suffering via medical beliefs or a practitioner's statements'.

***What, in reality, is reversible about the medicalized 'gender-affirming-care' pathway?***

There have also been claims that these procedures are reversible; indeed, naming a boy with a girl's name, or cross-dressing, is reversible. When, however, that pathway leads to drugs which atrophy sexual organs or surgeries that turn a male organ into the shape of a female organ, or vice versa, the moment of reversibility has passed. Never mind the removing of healthy breasts, the thinning of the vagina owing to the administration of hormones and the general neglect of follow up studies on the young people who have gone through these clinics, especially in the UK, but also in America. Is there a similar lack of follow up studies in other countries? At the same time, it has to be asked, how did WPATH, in 1979, become an expert in a phenomenon which had not yet found its way to the

free marketplace of ideas as the best means for discovering truth." Chiles, 146 S. Ct. at 1029.'

[17] "Iatrogenesis": https://en.wikipedia.org/wiki/Iatrogenesis.

gender clinics until the conjunction of Covid, mobile phones and, in the early 2000s, the dramatic escalation of young people, many of whom were young girls, thinking that they are "trans"?

The title of this book, then, includes the words, 'Transitioning from Health to Infertility'. Clearly, however, there is no guarantee that, ordinarily, what appear to be healthy sexual organs, will mean that the person will actually be fertile; and, therefore, this is not so much about being certain about fertility as not damaging what is, evidently, the natural expression of being male or female. Thus, in reality, if infertility does arise in the course of growing up it will necessarily need to be investigated and can range from overtiredness to more complicated causes. By contrast, however, if healthy sexual organs are mutilated in the course of producing a facsimile of the organs of the opposite sex, those same organs are actually and definitely rendered infertile.

Therefore, "Transitioning" is, in effect, passing from a state of health to a mutilated sexuality. This is not to say that there are not problems, of a mixed psychological, even physiological kind, about how to navigate puberty. But it is to say that there are parameters to physical interventions, given that healthy organs do not need to be mutilated, and that accompanying a person through growing up difficulties could well require specialist help of some kind and, without being too narrow, it could include both psychiatric help and the spiritual help of a minister. Nevertheless, in order that the discussion of what can help is well founded, it is also necessary to be very realistic about seeing the "whole" picture, with respect to each person, male or female, who presents. The whole picture includes, too, the prevalence of propaganda for gender ideology which has been percolating through clinics, schools, books, health service advice, police targeting gender critical comments, and the general targeting of gender critical academics.

So, with respect to a possible study on young people "electing" into a hormonal trial, how can the target group of this puberty blocker study be said to be "electing" into this study[18] when, already, there is such a pervasive mentality of persuasion in favour of it? Not least, when it comes to influential "others", is whether or not the school, clinicians, parents, and indeed peers are all pro-transitioning or, at the least, calling an adolescent's questioning of his or her sexuality an indication of being "in the wrong body". In other words, is there a serious, and conscientious, examination of the candidate that can "sift" these disposing factors while, at the same time, being critical and objective about any hormonal treatment procedure?[19] Never mind the prospect of surgical intervention. In other words, as we now know, the use of pronouns, how a person dresses, can all contribute to a path from "ideas" to a surgically impoverished sexuality.

## Previously published work

In a word, whether we draw on many authors or few, we are always drawing on what other people have found out; but, at the same time, each writer has his or her own provenance. To indicate this, I acknowledge my own background. Thus the following titles are now

---

[18] Cf. also Eleanor Hayward, June 19th, 2026, "NHS puberty blocker trial to go ahead for children as young as 11: https://archive.ph/w4BNL.

[19] Note the discussion of Judge Strum's remarks in *Transgenderism Two: Evidence and Identity*: https://enroutebooksandmedia.com/transgenderismtwo/.

on Amazon, in production or, as with this book, in the process of completion. I list them here in three groups: Scripture, theology, and philosophy; Bioethics; and autobiographical works; indeed, the third group began with a prayer in front of the Lady Chapel at our local Catholic Church, in the hope of writing a more widely accessible read.

Scripture: A Unique Word (2014); A trilogy on Faith and Reason called, From Truth and truth: Volume I-Faithful Reason (2016), Volume II-Faith and Reason in Dialogue (2016), Volume III-Faith is Married Reason (2016).

A second section of work, then, focuses on primarily bioethical questions. The Human Person: A Bioethical Word (2017), which endeavours to look at a person as a whole: as a concrete entity. Conception: An Icon of the Beginning (2019) is a monumental study of many aspects of questions concerning the definition of the beginning of each human person: of there being a first instant. Mary and Bioethics: An Exploration (2020), both begins to look at Mary's Immaculate Conception as entailing a first instant of ensoulment and holiness and, therefore, its illumination of each human conception; and, in addition, this book reaches more into the culture in which we live and, discovering transgenderism, reflects on various accounts and sources of it. Reaching for the Resurrection: A Pastoral Bioethics (2020), examines a number of bioethical questions more briefly, including the controversy around brain death: Can the person be dead if the body is alive? Unfolding a Post-Roe World (2022) opens up the possibility of the American Constitution being able to defend human life from conception and, in the course of doing so, provides a range of arguments that express the view that each of us is a person from the first instant of human conception. Human Nature: Moral Norm (2023), explores how being open to life is actually a more faithful account of the fullness of human nature. The *National Catholic Bioethics Centre* of America invited a contribution to Volume Two of a book on *Human Embryo Adoption: Catholic Arguments for and against*; my contribution is called "The Annunciation and Embryo Adoption" and argues that embryo adoption is a Marian participation in the saving work of Jesus Christ (2025).

While the following two books have autobiographical elements, as do most other books, they are more about the situation of our times than personal experience and, therefore, they warrant being in this section. The Word in Your Heart: Mary, Youth, and Mental Health (2024) is again drawing on the many studies of the problems that exist in our society and, particularly with respect to the youth, the need for ongoing philosophical and Christian formation. Transgenderism: A Question of Identity (2025), ranges over our society and comes to a gradual focus on transgenderism, which has turned up, little by little, in earlier work and begins to be the focus of more work. However, already, there is the pattern emerging of the rise of mobile phones, gender ideologist activists, and young people calling themselves "trans". Francis Etheredge, together with Elizabeth Rex, co-authored The Zygote of Christ and the Mystery of Man (2025); this book draws on very different essays by both authors, each of which contribute to a better understanding of the mystery of our beginning and the possibilities for doctrinal clarity from recent Church documents and legislative help for the unborn. Now Transgenderism Two: Evidence and Identity (2026), examines more deeply the recent documentation from the Supreme Court of the

United Kingdom on the 2010 Equality Act, a Report on Paediatric Medicine from America, and a Family Court Judgement from Australia, along with other material. What then follows, in this section, is a summary book on the major work which has been published up to now in this collection, called A Shorter Bioethics (2025). The Salvation of the Embryonic Person: Beginning with the Incarnation and the Immaculate Conception (2026), is a very focused study on following God's initiative: that if God began with the Incarnation, the conception of Christ from the first instant of His human conception, then this is the right place for us to reflect on His work of salvation. But there is also, the almost complete A New Way of Conceiving Conception, which strives for both a shorter and simpler account of accumulated research and work on the beginning of each one of us while, at the same time, giving prominence to the argument that there is a very first instant of human conception: of a personal presence from the first instant of fertilization (2026). In addition, there is this book, Transgenderism Three: Transitioning is From Health to Infertility (2026).

The third section of work is much more autobiographical and covers a variety of life events: The Family on Pilgrimage: God Leads Through Dead Ends (2018). The Prayerful Kiss: A Collection of Poetry and Prose (2019). Honest Rust and Gold: A Second Collection of Prose and Poetry (2020). Within Reach of You: A Book of Prose and Prayers (2021). Lord, Do You Mean Me? A father-Catechist!" (2023). An Unlikely Gardener: A Book of Prose and Poetry (2023). And now Time! Ladies and Gentlemen – Thoughts on Last Things (2025 – 2026). Meanwhile, I am now working on another book in this group called God is in the Detail: An Autobiography of a Pilgrim (2026-2027).

In summary, our life passes through many phases and difficulties and, while it is goal orientated to the fullness of life, we encounter more and more deeply the discovery of the necessity of God's help. And God's help is not just in a moment, which is when it concretely comes, but in the ongoing work of the word of God, the sacraments and the call to a new way of life through the living liturgy of the Church. In particular, there is the many mysterious promptings of the Holy Spirit and the redemptive and healing love of Jesus Christ, both of which constantly renews us individually and makes life with others more and more possible and fruitful. Thus, although these works are not explicitly bioethical, they are about the fullness of life to which we are called and which includes many dead ends and tragic turns; but, as one title says: "God Leads Through Dead Ends". Thus a boy who tried to commit suicide at thirteen or fourteen, ran away and came back, was asked to leave home twice, and who went through many crises, is now 70 years old, married for nearly thirty years, and a father of 11 children and an author of numerous books.

This work is about giving a foundation to what it means to be a person and, in terms of gender ideology, it is about showing what is being done to undo the mentality which leads to undoable harm. But hope is not optimism, it is a gift beyond our efforts and, therefore, everyone is invited to seek the help of the wounded healer, who is Jesus Christ.

The structure of this short book, then, begins with a summary overview of what passing through the questioning years is like for a real person. Then there is a very direct statement of what happens at the culmination of a process that begins with changing pronouns, names, using an invented language for what are familiar and well-founded realities, like being male or female, girl or boy, man or woman, husband or wife, or a mother or a father. But, first, in the next chapter, let us consider some of the general characteristics of growing up. However, even if the example of growing up is not typical, nevertheless, it illustrates the variety of "ideas of self" that a person can progress through until, as it were, the man or woman comes across what can be called "firm ground". Finally, this book concludes with a direct questioning of the need for any further research on the use of puberty blockers or any other kind of medication or surgical intervention in this field and a postscript on the American Federal case against WPATH and WPATH's reply.

# PART I

## THE QUESTIONING YEARS

If the people who help the youth, study the youth, what will they find? They may find a few people who know what they want to do and are motivated to do it. But, in general, according to the number of crises young people go through, or are in the midst of, it is clear that many enter upon adult life muddled in their thinking and, perhaps impatiently, hang out for certainties that are actually uncertain; and, therefore, have to spend time both unravelling their absorption in an interest or issue and, simultaneously, form a good understanding of life in the process. Whether a young person will meet God, is a bit of a mystery but, at the same time, I hope that they do not cling to false gods and, at the very least, search for the truth.

> Adapting what has been said elsewhere, 'we wish first of all to say to every person who is struggling: you are not alone. God loves you. Jesus never turned away those who suffered. He drew near to them, listened to them, touched them, restored their dignity, and brought them back into the community. The Church is called to do the same today. The Church loves you'[1].

---

[1] MOST REV. GILBERT A. GARCERA, D.D., Archbishop of Lipa, President, Catholic Bishops' Conference of the Philippines. 13th July, 2026, "Come to me, all you who labour and are burdened: CBCP pastoral letter on mental health, compassion, and hope": https://cbcpnews.net/cbcpnews/cbcp-pastoral-letter-on-mental-health-compassion-and-hope/.

***If the search for self is the goal, how common is the experience of shedding many provisional ideas until we identify ourselves wholly?***

Having entered adolescence without any clear idea of what I wanted to do, I went through any number of ideas, including thinking that, in my late teens, it would be easier if I was a woman, as I would not have to work all this out. I somehow had the idea that a woman did not have to work out who she was; it was somehow self-evident that she would marry and be at home[2]. In other words, I was just as ignorant about a woman's identity as I was about my own; after all, both my mother and all my sisters came to recognize their talents, went on to train and, also, to marry.

As for myself, I went through so many ideas of what I wanted to be that it would read like stations on the circle line and, in the end, I came back to the person I began with, namely, myself. One image which has remained with me, covering many years, was that travelling was like always disturbing the water and never letting it become like a mirror. As I had started to seek advice, at a certain point I was

---

[2] Similarly, Stella O'Malley, a psychotherapist, recognizes that, when growing up, she would have "swiped' puberty blockers 'from your hand" but now leads evidence-based opposition to gender ideology; Rachel Baxendale, July 20th, 2026, "Leading therapist claims a 'different level of fear' gags Australia's gender debate: As a gender-distressed child, psychotherapist Stella O'Malley says she would have 'swiped' puberty blockers 'from your hand'. Now she's leading an international battle against medicalisation": https://archive.md/2026.07.19-204845/https://www.theaustralian.com.au/nation/leading-therapist-claims-a-different-level-of-fear-gags-australias-gender-debate/news-story/5a6549f027f60b219128cb2dbde117a7.

advised, to use an image, to scoop up some water in a bowl and, when it settled, to look in the mirror and remember what I saw. My first attempt to stop travelling lasted less than three years and then I managed five in a big city where, while dropping out of one course, and completing others, I eventually began studying what has become a life-long study of Scripture, theology, and philosophy, with a focus on contemporary culture.

### *Writing an investigation begins with investigating writing*

The question that dominated so many years of my life was: What am I going to do? The answer that began to take shape involved recognizing that failing to complete a psychology degree, dropping out of a teaching course, not getting onto a music degree, taking a Foundation course in Fine Art but going no further, redoing 'A' levels and ending up with 7, 6 of which involved written work, plus a Certificate in Religious Education, all of which involved writing. Thus the very nature of the courses that I was doing began to point towards being a writer. But to write about what? And so many possibilities burst like balloons, leaving a trail of debris that, in itself, was also a source of material that, in later years, was useful for writing and research. But, like a light from my childhood, one of the subjects that I had not tried was theology, which was that subject which was less than an 'A' level and which began a thirty-five-year love affair with theology, anthropology, and bioethics, and which is still ongoing!

### *Unbeknown to myself a writer*

In one sense, the desire to write was an unwelcome and unrecognized inclination. I can say this because I did not know what to do for many years. I tried many different subjects, many of which were writing based. However, coming from an artistic family, and failing many subjects at school, except one: Religious Education, I also failed to follow in my parents' footsteps either into art or more generally in knowing what I wanted to do. So, there were many years of doing things which did not, at first, turn me into a writer. Having said that, however, I did try to write in my twenties but having no computer, it was paper and glue, tippex, scissors and, literally, cutting and pasting. But the impossibility of finishing anything finished me off for a number of years. I mention all this because it became the raw material, as it were, out of which a lot of exploratory writing emerged. This led to various breakdowns, at different times, one landing me in a psychiatric ward for several weeks in my twenties. So, not knowing what I wanted to do entailed many journeys, trying out many courses, types of work, and even a relatively long period as a self-employed maintenance man; but it also involved going for spiritual guidance and trying out different lives, as it were, by visiting priests and monks and sharing a little of what went on in parishes and monasteries. Thus, although I wrote a lot it was mainly essays, with long breaks in between and then, after abandoning various courses, I began to settle on theology. It was as if, having tried so many fruitless options, a lighted candle came out of my past, from my early school days, and like a light in the darkness started a program of courses which went on for some twenty-five plus years, on and off until, eventually, I was able to leave paid work and write full-time.

In the course of these years was the related battle with sexuality; and, like David who withdrew from the battle while his army was at war, so I withdrew from the battle and suffered similarly. A woman with whom I had a child went and aborted him or her. Thus there emerged the question of when does a person's life begin, because that brief life had given me so much joy and pain?[3] Another question that arose from my experience was what makes contraception wrong? And then also: How is it possible to live the Christian life when, like a broken Christian, I kept losing the battle for chastity? These questions, then, in the course of many courses of study, began to develop into a number of book type investigations. I was even granted a thousand pounds to write a book by the Diocese of Birmingham but, trying to do it without taking advantage of the adviser I was given, it failed and took another twenty years to write; and, the final version, was more fully about being open to life. Similarly with the question of when a human life begins. Given my own experience of loss, I discovered an unanswered question in the teaching of the Catholic Church, namely when, precisely does a human life begin? And, again, this set me on a path for another book that also took around twenty years to write. More widely, then, there is a mixture of life experience coming together with many years of theological and scriptural study, each complementing the other, and together these sources acted like yeast amongst the dough, and so many books came forth in this way - perhaps all of them, some more directly and others more indirectly drawing on personal experience. This even applies

---

[3] Cf. "Indelible", in the Prayerful Kiss: https://enroutebooksandmedia.com/theprayerfulkiss/.

to my experience of marriage, fatherhood, our children being home for covid, all eight of them, and many many pilgrimages.

As regards formative influences, I remember once seeing St. John Paul II on television when he came to England and I, at the time, was not anything in particular, although I had been brought up Catholic and was in and out of Churches like one going in and out of a rotating door. Nevertheless when, at around 35, I started studying theology, I began to gravitate to the teaching of the popes and particularly the work of St. John Paul II. His work was a very formative influence; and, in many ways, laid a foundation upon which I continue to build. Another, very formative influence, was coming into contact with the Neocatechumenal Way, which is a life-long way of adult formation in the faith. In the course of this way there were many experiences, including the discovery that I had no faith, had not changed, and was thrown out by the Gospel of the man who was at the wedding feast without changing his clothes. But, owing to returning to this way after my experience of reading the Catechism, I benefited from many counsels, sources of advice, sacraments of the Church and, as I say, many pilgrimages. So, although this was a pivotal experience, it was very simple. I had failed again to go beyond a "relationship" to marriage; and, my reaction, as I am now forty, was a hopelessness in which three possibilities surfaced: more sin; mental illness; and suicide. However, I was reading the *Catechism of the Catholic Church*, probably for an essay, and it said, 'If God can create everything out of nothing, he can make a new beginning for the sinner' (paragraph 298). No one spoke, there was no unusual event, and I do not know how it even happened – but I know that after reading those lines everything changed. Because of those lines, I returned to the

Neocatechumenal Way, went on pilgrimage and, within a year, married and have been married for going on thirty years.

Perhaps the last influence, to be concise, is reading very widely and discovering a number of crises in our culture, each with an echo, as it were, in my own life. In other words, the more social commentary I have read the more I realise that a lot of my struggles and sufferings are shared by so many. But, now, I am able to draw upon so. many gifts and graces of God. So, two of the most recent books are about the problems of youth, gender ideology, and the contribution of many kinds of scholarship in conjunction with the help of the word of God.

***Common threads: Who am I and who are we?***

My very first writings were about exploring the stream of consciousness account of being myself; and, unfortunately, I no longer have them, having abandoned them to the scrap heap. But, it is possible to say that these early writings, which were not essays for courses, were about responding to questions: How do I give an account of what is going on in my life? What do we know about the beginning of each one of us? Why is there so much destruction of human life? My letters to newspapers, even Catholic newspapers or journals, might occasionally get published; indeed, one essay on being a student in my thirties, did actually get published in the Catholic Times. The theme, then, of giving an account of my life entails an autobiographical impulse, one might say, which has been there from very early on. But so, too, is writing as a vehicle of investigation: When does each one of us begin? Amidst, then, of any number of courses, there was always this impulse to write about what struck me as interesting and invaluably true; and, as my first Course Director said: I was not the best student – but he thought I had something to say. Thus, that impulse to "say something", has never left me completely even if, at times, I fear it has been exhausted.

The very early books were long and somewhat called out of years of writing, either because of writing essays or because a question had started me off on a path of research. So, the mystery of Scripture, its capacity to influence an investigation, to prompt questions and research, and to "cause" a change, was a book to counter the claim that Scripture is a quasi-historical account that may or may not be true but is certainly desiccated by innumerable scholars into a book barely worth reading in that almost, line by line, the question was not does God speak and act, but who wrote it and what were the subsequent changes by later authors. In other words, Scripture has a power to change lives and prompt research; indeed, it is both about the change that God "caused" in the history of salvation and, therefore, the change that God can continue to cause in the present. This is because the nature of the word of God is that it is a truly human and divine word; it is not a human word made divine: it is intrinsically and inseparably a human and a divine word (cf. *Dei Verbum*[4]). On the human level, we can experience the power of a naturally human word; and so, for example, owing to repression, not just forgetfulness, I lost the humiliations I experienced at school and my entire history with it, up until I started searching for what I did not

[4] There are a lot of Church documents which attest to the mystery of the word of God; *Dei Verbum* is from the Second Vatican Council, but Pope Benedict wrote *Verbum Domini* etc.

remember but knew, as it were, my memories were missing. One night, restless, I had a kind of waking dream and imagined shaking some kind of creature off my hand and then a dam breaking, the kind of dam I built many times in my childhood on the beach and, following on from that, my whole hidden history flowed back until, as it were, it ran like the stream of consciousness that it was intended to do. On the divine level, then, a word of God has the power to bring about what is beyond my power to do so; and so, as I have mentioned, God gave me faith in His existence and that He helps, without me even realizing, very clearly, that I was completely bereft of faith: that it was dead. Thus, the word of God, has a unique power[5] to illuminate our lives and to help us.

This echoes the mystery of the *Incarnation*: Jesus Christ is truly human and truly divine; he is not a man made divine: Christ is truly, and inseparably, both human and divine. Similarly, the Church is both human and divine (*Lumen Gentium*, 8[6]); and, indeed, each of the sacraments of the Church express this uniquely: the words said, the water poured, and the action of the Holy Spirit constitute the mystery of Baptism: an outward sign of an inner action of God. In other words, the mystery of the word of God is a mystery which, like leaven, can come into whatever we do. Grace and nature interact, complement each other, and continue the creative work of the Creator. Thus it is always about drawing on the interrelationship between

---

[5] The book dedicated to this subject is called "Scripture: A Unique Word": https://www.cambridgescholars.com/product/978-1-4438-6044-4; but, given that the word of God is a living word, it is referred to throughout my collected works; cf. the En Route Books and Media published website: https://enroutebooksandmedia.com/francisetheredge/.

[6] This is also a document of the Second Vatican Council on the Church.

what is natural and what is supernatural, what is from nature and what is from grace, such that a "holistic" account of reality takes account of both as, in the end, God is the author of both nature and grace and the two, therefore, as the Church constantly teacher, are inseparable in the work of salvation.

Whatever the subject of the writing, then, it is always about what do we know about ourselves, as human beings, being male or female, and called to relationship: that relationship is a theme of God's creation is expressed in all that the Creator does. Whether through evidence, reason, observation, previous work, experience, the word of God, theology, philosophy, or culture, we are called to answer that call of God. But simultaneously, it is always about searching out what is true, either because truth will not contradict truth, or because truth is actually a goal in itself; indeed, I would call the human person a truth seeker: just as a dog can follow a scent, or an arrow arrive at a target even if there is an impossible number of stops in between, so human beings are built to be "truth-seekers". We are "truth-seekers" about ourselves, or we are lost, as we are "truth-seekers" about anything that exists; the truth is the magnetic north to which, even if we are disorientated at times, we are constantly called to find. But the "magnetic north" is both what really exists: what "is"; and the magnetic north is a person, is God, and so it is not so much that we seek, as that we follow a lead, a trail, an indication of where to go and what awaits to be discovered. Moreover, what we discover has to draw upon how we can communicate our discoveries to others; indeed, as another has said, our task is to communicate "heart to heart".

But, as we are social beings, the desire is to be in communion, and so to foster that common recognition of what is true which builds human community; and, ultimately, to realize that we are founded on God as the origin, the way, and the goal of all our activity: the Love that elicits love. Just as God is a communion of three, in that he is the Blessed Trinity: three persons in one God - so we are many but called to be one in Christ's redeeming love of us.

Even if we do not all proceed evenly on the path of truth; it is nevertheless necessary that there is a common starting point that structures our social interactions, and which is expressed in law, medicine, education and society's many groups or we end up just dissolving into endless disputes. Are we reaching the point where there are those who are more for "dispute" than for the common good?

***As we proceed, so there emerges other sources to assist us***

In a pastoral letter on mental health, although written for a particular jurisdiction, it picks up on a number of common threads throughout this research on mental health and young people, noting its increase, but adding that it is not a 'sign of weak faith' or 'a punishment for sin' but is a condition that 'deserves understanding, appropriate care, and compassionate accompaniment.' At the same time this letter notes the whole context of what impacts young people, including the social situation, the presence of the media, and the possibility of losing hope[7]. Although then, this letter does not

---

[7] ✠ MOST REV. GILBERT A. GARCERA, D.D., Archbishop of Lipa, President, Catholic Bishops' Conference of the Philippines. 13th July, 2026, "Come to me, all you who labour and are burdened: CBCP pastoral letter on mental health,

mention gender ideology, it nevertheless refers to 'other threats to mental well-being'[8].

By way of another confirmation of an increasingly widespread view, a recent report on young people, particularly, has highlighted both a common characteristic of growing up and the help of faith communities. However, while 'Religious communities' cannot be understood uncritically, the following report confirms a widespread sense that young people, and maybe their parents too, are increasingly vulnerable to the extent that they are not developing a coherent world view or philosophy of life, the lack of which makes them particularly susceptible to "belonging" to activist groups which give them ready made, but "monosyllabic" answers to what is going on in their lives and in the world today.

> 'Childhood and adolescence are not merely periods in which individuals acquire skills; they are also stages in which they seek a stable answer to the question of who they are and where they belong. Religious communities can provide shared practices, intergenerational relationships, moral reference points and a narrative that places personal suffering within a wider horizon of meaning'[9].

---

compassion, and hope": https://cbcpnews.net/cbcpnews/cbcp-pastoral-letter-on-mental-health-compassion-and-hope/.

[8] Gilbert A. Garcera, "Come to me, all you who labour and are burdened."

[9] JORGE ENRIQUE MÚJICA, July 22nd, 2026, "Less religion in childhood, poorer mental health in adolescence: what the results of a scientific study show": https://zenit.org/2026/07/22/less-religion-in-childhood-poorer-mental-health-in-adolescence-what-the-results-of-a-scientific-study-show/?eti=34375.

> Thus 'Material well-being can alleviate many forms of suffering, but it cannot by itself answer questions about identity, belonging, purpose or the place of the individual within a larger moral community'[10].

People need a sound formation in both thinking and the reality of the Christian faith, including the fact that God acts in the history of salvation and continues to act in our lives and, at the same time, invites us to seek to be welcomed by our Mother, the Church, drawing us into a relationship with Christ.

---

[10] MÚJICA, July 22nd, 2026, "Less religion in childhood, poorer mental health in adolescence: what the results of a scientific study show".

# PART II

## QUESTIONS HAVE ANSWERS

Although crises are very challenging at the time, it is possible that there is a benefit to having to work through any number of real-life questions which are both very personal and, at the same time, very prevalent in society. In other words, there is a benefit to having to think through questions of personal identity, the nature of human personhood, personal experience, and the *pros* and *cons* of the medicalization of the crises that we go through. What is that benefit? That a writer and a researcher is not obliged to follow a school of thought but, rather, to follow where the truth leads, whether it is to evidence, to philosophy, or to the nature of religious faith.

***How did these investigations begin?***

After gender ideology surfaced in a book discussing the mystery of Mary, the *Mother of God*, it became clear that gender ideology was a recurring subject in a variety of surveys of what goes on in contemporary society, particularly because it seeks to dissolve the distinction between being male and female. This endeavour to dissolve the binary sex distinction of being male or female, the more it is excavated, the deeper the roots run back into the past and the thought of the radical feminists who not only wanted to abolish the family but, in order to abolish the family, also wanted to deny the reality of the two sexes too. Now, there are two particularly focused books on refuting the transgenderist claim: the claim that sex is transferable from boy to girl, from girl to boy, or from man to woman or woman to man. The first book was about the general malaise in society, noting the rise of mental health problems, suicide, the rise of social media and its take up by the young. Then the book gravitated, more and more, to the questions which were arising from what was happening in gender clinics; and, therefore, the wide-spreading questioning of what is a boy or a girl? What is a man or a woman? And are there real differences between boys and girls, men and women? This book also began to address the discovery that when philosophy and Christian theology disappear from a culture, so the vacuum can be filled by many other things, all of which show that people are increasingly incapable of assessing the reality of gender ideology. Thus, this first book also examines the many helps to those who are caught up in ideas that trap people in impossible choices, and the extent to which gender ideology is impervious to criticism, demonizing counselling, and pillorying opposition. Addressing the situation, then, not only needs clear thinking but prayer, research and an increasing grasp of the anthropology of gift: that each of us is a gift: we receive the gift of our being – from both our parents and from God.

The second book, building on the first one, was even more focused on the whole subject of the identity of a woman as, in a very particular way, boys and men were claiming to be girls and women. Thus these book began to discover, and to show, the widespread influence of gender ideology, particularly at the United Nations and in innumerable institutions throughout the western world, while also seeking to impose that same ideology on nations dependent on western aid. Furthermore, the second book examines three more major documents, having begun in the course of the first one to examine the rise of social media and the Cass Report on gender clinics in the UK. The second book, then, continues with a more specific focus on the incoherence of gender ideology itself. At the same time, it is clear that so insidious is the language of gender ideology that, inadvertently, even those documents criticising it, use the gender ideologists' incorrect biological concepts, such that sex is determined at birth[1]. What is more, even a recent, American Supreme Court judgement, has drawn upon the claim that sex is determined at birth[2], which is

---

[1] Cf. Etheredge, *Transgenderism Two: Evidence and Identity*: https://enroutebooksandmedia.com/transgenderismtwo/.

[2] Cf. Judge Sotomayor, pages 1-33, and Judge Jackson's comments pp. 1-3, where the pages refer to their own contributions to their opinions and not to the page numbers of the whole document. The case is: "WEST VIRGINIA ET AL. v. B. P. J., BY HER NEXT FRIEND AND MOTHER, HEATHER JACKSON CERTIORARI TO THE UNITED STATES COURT OF APPEALS FOR THE FOURTH CIRCUIT", No. 24–43. Argued January 13, 2026—Decided June 30, 2026: https://www.supremecourt.gov/opinions/25pdf/24-43_2b35.pdf. There are a number of problems here: the notable use of gender ideology terminology, by Sotomayor, 'cisgender' for an actual girl, the idea that sex is determined at birth, which it is not, sex is determined at conception, and Sotomayor's constant use of the pronoun 'she' for the boy. Nowhere in the judgements of the judges is 'biological sex' defined; however, Sotomayor refers to 'sex identified at birth' (p. 2) and so does Jackson, too (pp. 1-3); and, in addition, Jackson also uses the gender ideology terms, too, namely 'a cisgender woman'. The problem with defining biological sex as sex at birth is that this is not a biological definition of sex: sex is defined by chromosomes, the type of reproductive cells, male and female, and the psychosomatic whole of the individual man or woman. 'Cisgender', then, is an unnecessary word, as it is a word coined to mean 'a person whose gender identity corresponds with the sex registered for them at birth; not transgender': https://google.com/search?q=cisgender+meaning Therefore, 'cisgender' is simply referring to a boy or a girl, from conception, and registered when recognized, whether at birth or earlier and, as such, using a prefix to indicate 'on the side of' and, in addition, is replacing sex, male or female, with a word with a particular agenda and with its own controversial history and use: "Cisgender": https://en.wikipedia.org/wiki/Cisgender.

biologically inaccurate. Sex is determined by the combination of chromosomes at conception, manifesting, progressively, in the outward male and female reproductive organs, and the physiological and hormonal prompts, long before puberty, which structure the person as male or female. Puberty confirms, unfolds more fully, and intimately expresses the psychological completion of the maturing man or woman. The point being that a man or a woman is a whole being, a whole person, and not some kind of self-chosen combination of parts. Each of us is a whole gift, unique, and unrepeatable; but, in being so, we are either a male or a female human person.

***The law, terminology, and debate: Two types of gender ideologists***

> *In Norway, children "decide" their legal sex from the age of six, with one parent in agreement, while parents risk up to six years' imprisonment if they fail to comply with their child's declared "gender identity".*[3]

While Norway seems to have lost its objectivity almost completely, other countries are in different stages or degrees of ideological indoctrination. Those who advocate gender ideology and who are incapable of a critical appreciation of it, are a distinct group, possibly untrained in child psychology, and ideologically incapable of escaping the narrative of historical injustice and claiming "victimization" or "transphobia", "against" anyone who is critical of this ideology. The

---

[3] Anne Kalvig, August 29th, 2026, "Gender Identity: A Religious Belief Treated as Reality": https://jbilek.substack.com/p/gender-identity-a-religious-belief.

second book, then, goes on to discuss the philosophical world view which seems, more and more, to be basically anti-life, anti-population, and anti-Christian, manipulating facts into a "hypothetically affirmative" narrative called 'gender affirming care'. This is "hypothetically affirmative" of young people who are thinking they are in the "wrong body" because the condition does not exist as an existential reality; rather, it is a construct of ideologists, which is then confirmed by clinicians who are incapable of examining the full, human reality, of the person who presents. A fact, for example, that some children are born with ambiguous genitalia, although not necessarily with ambiguous chromosomes, is then taken out of its biological context and turned into a supposed "third sex", which is not what this condition is; rather, ambiguous genitalia is a true clinical condition which needs careful analysis, and even delayed intervention, to see how the child develops. But it is certainly not a "third sex".

At the same time, using or rather misusing the law to silence debate and discussion, gender ideology has spread into sport, schools, anti-discrimination legislation and, in the end, "holds court" on what is good practice when, in reality, its ideologists are incapable of assessing their own claims objectively. What is therefore rather striking is that a prominent Australian psychiatrist, who's right to question a questionable treatment has been vindicated after four years, has yet been required, as it were, not to return to her previous position; and, indeed, is now under yet another investigation[4], which

---

[4] Mackenzie Scott, July 17th, 2026, "Queensland Children's Hospital clears psychiatrist over gender treatment concerns: Queensland Children's Hospital has formally cleared suspended Dr Jillian Spencer of wrongdoing, four years after she raised clinical concerns about gender treatment": https://archive.md/DOQhC.

gives the impression of an unrelenting use of the law against anyone who criticizes gender ideology[5]. So, one wonders, how valid is the claim that gender ideology will not determine the "one path" down which children will be sent: from pronouns to hormones to surgery?[6]

These cases are turning up, regularly, and are a constant challenge to the right to appreciate the reality of sex-based differences and the right of the female sex to their own sports and safe places[7].

---

[5] Stephen Rice, March 31st, 2026, "She shared a news story. Now she could lose her medical licence: Child psychiatrist Jillian Spencer faces an investigation after sharing an article from The Australian that quoted her concerns about gender-affirming treatment": https://archive.md/jvlx7#selection-661.0-665.161; cf. also Stephanie Bastiaan and Rachael Wong, December 10th, 2025, "The case of Kirralie Smith and how NSW's anti-vilification laws are being weaponised against women": https://www.womensforumaustralia.org/the_case_of_kirralie_smith_and_how_nsws_anti_vilification_laws_are_being_weaponised_against_women.

[6] Mackenzie Scott, July 17th, 2026, "Queensland Children's Hospital clears psychiatrist over gender treatment concerns.

[7] Cf. Even recently, Jackson Thompson, June 30th, 2026, "Supreme Court makes ruling on trans athletes in women's sports". Thus 'states have the right to designate sports teams based on biological sex, not gender identity': https://www.foxnews.com/sports/supreme-court-makes-ruling-trans-athletes-womens-sports. The case is: "WEST VIRGINIA ET AL. v. B. P. J., BY HER NEXT FRIEND AND MOTHER, HEATHER JACKSON CERTIORARI TO THE UNITED STATES COURT OF APPEALS FOR THE FOURTH CIRCUIT", No. 24–43. Argued January 13, 2026—Decided June 30, 2026: https://www.supremecourt.gov/opinions/25pdf/24-43_2b35.pdf. All references to page numbers refer to the individual justice's comments and not to the document as a whole. JUSTICE KAVANAUGH delivered the opinion of the Court, for the American Supreme Court, pp. 2-3, and says that: 'may schools determine eligibility for women's and girls' sports based on biological sex? The answer is yes.' Furthermore, on p. 7, the Court says: 'The law further found that the benefit "that natural testosterone provides to male athletes is not diminished through the use of puberty blockers and cross-sex hormones. §33–6202(11).' Indeed, the ruling continually refers to the original legislation, protecting and promoting female only sports, whereby female is defined by biological sex; and, indeed, is similar to the outcome of the UK

---

Supreme Court finding that the terms of the Equality Act of 2010 referred to biological males and biological females. At the same time, this ruling very reasonably articulates the injustice to females if males, irrespective of their additional hormone input, compete against females. By contrast, the case for the boy who identifies as a girl, defended by JUSTICE SOTOMAYOR, rests on the view that there is a commensurate "equality" between the boy identifying as a girl and girls, owing to the lack of 'endogenous puberty' in the boy and the effect of additional hormones and who, therefore, "should" be allowed to participate in actual girls' sports (pp. 1-33). Sotomayor, however trustingly, assumes that the boy's identification as a girl is his true identity. In other words, Sotomayor is playing into the fiction that the boy can be a girl and, it seems, is basing this on no more than the boy's claim and what it has led to in terms of his receiving hormones and the whole legal appeal through the courts. In other words, Sotomayor is not capable of perceiving the possibility that the boy, like 90-95% of such children, will be reconciled to his sex at conception. Moreover, even those not resolved have to be investigated from the point of view of their longevity, the influence of pro-gender ideology activists, and other factors. Sotomayor becomes one more influential adult who endorses the fiction of a true sex change and contributes, as Cass says, to an irreversible consequence for his adult, male sexuality. The value of Sotomayor's contribution is her emphasis on the individuality of the boy who identifies as a girl; however, Sotomayor's perception of the boy's individuality does not take account of the possibility that the boy is mistaken about his identity and will revert, later, and even regret his use of hormones, however sanctioned by others, leading to whatever damage to his fertility it may already have caused or may still cause (*ibid*). As regards Sotomayor's legal scrutiny of the majority judgment, it has some interesting points to make with respect to the impact of Trump's Executive Order on the rejection of transgender athletes not competing in any other than their original sex category (*ibid*); however, the majority judgement cites a lot of common evidence on the difference between male and female sporting capabilities although, in general, these are characteristics not true of every individual male or female but are appropriately relevant to sport, wherein men and woman train specifically to enhance their capabilities. In sum, however, the court does not deprive the boy of the wonderful benefits of sport (cf. Sotomayor, p. 33); and, typically, we are left with an emotional argument which seeks to manipulate others rather than to address the boy's particular difficulties which, in general, were never discussed or investigated nor was it suggested that counselling might help him, although Judge Thomas does refer to this himself (p. 2 of his comments). Although, contrary to

Indeed, in contrast to the recent court judgements in America and the United Kingdom, each of which has recognized the definition of a man or a woman according to their sex, however imperfectly by referring to their sex at birth, an Australian court is still labouring under the confusion of including men in their definition of women:

> Although, as some contend, it seems largely unintended, the decoupling of the definition of man and woman from biological sex, 'by removing the explicit biological definitions of a man and a woman, the Act has since been interpreted by the courts as preferencing gender identity ahead of biological sex'.
>
> 'The issue is central to the Tickle v Giggle court case where the Federal Court has ruled the Sex Discrimination Act [amended in 2013[8]] does not confine the legal concept of sex to biological sex, and found that Sall Grover's company, Giggle, which was designed for women, had

---

considering what will actually help the boy, Sotomayor seems to think that being allowed to play on a girls' team will help (p. 33).

In general, Sotomayor and Jackson lack the critical scrutiny evinced by Judge Strum in Australia (cf. Etheredge, Transgender Two: Evidence and Identity). And, more widely, the assumption that 'biological sex' means 'sex assigned at birth' is not biological sex; biological sex is just that: sex at conception, which unfolds anatomically; physiologically; and psychosomatically in terms of being male or female, boy or girl, man or woman. Man or woman being the natural goal of the whole process, unfolding from conception, continuously, and uninterruptedly. This is not a discussion of medical disorders and therefore applies generally.

[8] Cf. Sall Grover, May 19th, 2026, "I will never be lectured on misogyny by Julia Gillard, and neither should you: While the former PM continues to lecture the world on what it means to be a woman in public life, I am left dealing with her disastrous legacy": https://archive.md/z9NIf#selection-673.0-677.144.

discriminated against trans woman Roxanne Tickle [who is a man] on the basis of appearance'[9]. Since when is being a man, or a woman, for that matter, based on appearance? In other words, it is not intrinsically discriminatory to recognize that a man is a man even if he claims to be a woman.

Again, in Queensland, the litigation that proceeds, it seems, interminably, centres on what is real: Is there an equivalence between an actual woman breastfeeding and a man chest-feeding? What drugs are literally expressed in a man chest-feeding a child? Are those drugs harmful? Is there justice to the child to be the object of an experimental practice?[10] Why cannot these questions be discussed without interminable legal proceedings?[11]. Again, there seems to be an abandonment of objective evidence which, actually, includes the well-known and established goodness of a mother's milk (not withstanding exceptional problems with it which, in general, are generally treatable).

In the case of the proposed legislation for New Zealand, which is not about discrimination or denying variations in actual people; rather, it is about clarifying the law: 'The

---

[9] Rachel Baxendale, Jacquelin Magnay and Elizabeth Pike, "'It was a different time': Julia Gillard remark ignites push on gender law": https://archive.md/WDd7H#selection-1697.0-1697.74.

[10] Cf. Ameer Kotecha, August 2nd, 2026, "We need a crackdown on crackpot charities": https://spectator.com/article/we-need-a-crackdown-on-crackpot-charities/.

[11] Human Rights Law Alliance, June 26th, 2026, "Jasmine Sussex returns to Brisbane tribunal as vilification case continues": https://www.hrla.org.au/j asmine-sussex-returns-to-brisbane-tribunal-as-vilification-case-continues.

> Legislation (Definitions of Woman and Man) Amendment Bill, introduced by Marcroft, passed its first reading last month.
>
> The bill would amend the Legislation Act 2019 by adding a definition of "woman" as "an adult human biological female" and of "man" as "an adult human biological male"'"[12].

Ultimately, the law has to use language that communicates reality; otherwise, the law is evincing a philosophically unsound claim with widespread ramifications, namely, that the law is "independent" of reality.

Thus, apart from those gender ideological activists already referred to, there is a second group, namely those doctors, surgeons, clinicians, psychiatrists, lawyers, politicians, and parents and indeed, young or older young people, who have come out of this "ideological thought clothing and cloning", and have started to see how destructive, uncritical, unreal, unprofessional, and really harmful gender ideology actually is. In this category there are those who, within the WPATH organisation, seem to be trying to think through the discrepancies in their ideology; and, therefore, are wondering how people who have gone through with irreversible changes can be helped. But, at the same time, there does not seem to be the freedom to think that irreversible changes are to be publicized and avoided. Nevertheless, one response went almost this far:

---

[12] Hannah McCallum, June 30th, 2026, "'I'm not a scientist': MP defends sex definition bill that omits intersex Kiwis": https://newsroom.co.nz/ 2026/06/30/im-not-a-scientist-nz-first-mp-defends-sex-definition-bill-that-omits-intersex-kiwis/?utm_medium=Social&utm_source=LinkedIn#Echobox=1782847351-1.

> 'Marci Bowers, a highly influential transgender surgeon and former president of WPATH, called the patient's situation "tragic" and wrote that one of WPATH's great challenges was to "help patients sort through their gender diverse feelings" before receiving "irreversible treat-ment."[13] In other words, it does not look as if WPATH has reached the conclusion that 'irreversible changes' are in themselves a limit too far; and, indeed, one voice proposed that sometimes it is necessary to go too far: some 'people need to go 'too far' before they realize where they want to be'.

But again, this 'too far' is irreversible and is tantamount to absolving those who advise and action these irreversible changes of all responsibility for what has been done to a person who, in their inexperience of life, did not know they might change and regret the wholesale destruction of their sexual organs – while their sex remains unchanged to that of their original sex at conception. Another member of WPATH wondered if 'it might be helpful to educate young transgender patients seeking sex-change surgery on the "potential benefit" of keeping their ovaries, "just in case."'[14] More fundamentally, then, this kind of discussion reveals that WPATH does not

---

[13] Megan Brock, July 30th, 2026, "Inside WPATH: Trans Org Admits Need For Detransitioner Protocols While Pushing Child Sex-Changes": "There is a critical and undeniable need for detransitioner protocols — a reality acknowledged even by WPATH's own members": https://www.dailywire.com/ news/wpath-files-trans-org-admits-need-for-detransitioner-protocols-while-pushing-child-sex-changes.

[14] Megan Brock, July 30th, 2026, "Inside WPATH: Trans Org Admits Need for Detransitioner Protocols While Pushing Child Sex-Changes".

have the authority to claim that it is a leading authority in this field as these discussions reveal that people are at "sea" with the reality of what is being done, especially to young people, who may yet regret what is done to them. On the one hand, WPATH advocates serious, bodily changes to young people; and, on the other hand, WPATH is discovering its own inadequacy when it comes to addressing those same 'irreversible changes'. In other words, what is stopping WPATH recognizing that 'irreversible changes' are actually a harm: a harm that has been medically caused?

While, however, this gender ideology reigns in the courts, it will continue to cost enormous amounts of time and money, as well as risk the safety of young people, particularly girls and women; but, also, it calls the law into contempt as the law is patently using concepts that are "free floating" and not grounded in reality. The problem of the law not being grounded in reality, in an actual definition of man and woman which is independent of "ideological fashions", in and of itself unravels the nature of justice which entails a relationship to truth: to truth evidenced by common experience and standard science.

This third book, then, shorter than the rest, is really seeking to show, more briefly, not only the fruit of further research, but what makes the ideological mentality so naked, especially given the increasingly and widely published actual harms for which it is responsible.

# PART III

# THE STULTIFICATION OF DEVELOPMENT

In view, then, of my own psychological zigzagging through many years, types of courses, ideas of what I want to be, including many others that I have not referred to very much, such as being a musician, a lawyer, a doctor, a psychiatric nurse, and a footballer, it follows that anyone who has a real history will traverse many possibilities in the course of their growing up. The problem, then, is not so much change as that underlying change is constancy; and, indeed, life is about discovering that "keel": that basic structure of who one is and what is entailed in being me, you, or whoever. The deepest identity, the one at the root of being and inclusive of every other kind of good gift, whether that of being male or female, replete with talents, is that which expresses relationship: our relationship to each other and to God; and, given that it is often, if not always, that crises arise in our relationships, and impact the other areas of our life, it is essential to discover, indeed, to accept, that we are children of God called to be beings-in-relationship. Nevertheless, we can find ourselves down any number of labyrinthine pathways; however, however far we go from others and from God, we are never too far to be out of reach of both other people and God Himself. And, indeed, one of the greatest gifts of Christ to His Church is the gift of the *Sacrament of Reconciliation*: The possibility of recognizing that we have erred, sinned, gone astray, and that God forgives and helps us.

***Is there evidence that gender ideology leads to harm?***

What counts as evidence in an investigation can be approached in a number of ways. Certainly, evidence can be obtained from systematic reviews. These reviews, however, do not address the immediate consequence of a course of treatment and, what is more, there are long delays in actually accumulating enough data which, anyway, is subject to some kind of statistical analysis. In other words, systematic reviews do not address, directly, the immediate harm of a course of treatment. Nor do systematic reviews take into account the influence of a parent who wants to transition a child[1]. Nor does the review take account of the milieu within which a child self-declares that they are in the wrong body. Does the literature take account of whether or not there were proper psychiatric diagnoses, co-morbidities, or any other influential factors in the whole scenario leading up to the actual mutilations of the body of either a minor, young person, or adult? There are hormones, then, that thin the wall of the vagina, and which can lead to rupture and bleeding. There is the making of an artificial, facsimile, male organ into a facsimile of female hole in a boy's anatomy. In other words a healthy organ is mutilated and the child is left with a wound which has to be kept open. Or there is a kind of penis-like protrusion in a girl's anatomy mutilating, as with the boy, the natural sexual organ of the girl. Then there is, also, the victimization of people, whether medical professionals, lecturers,

[1] Cf. Judge Strum in Etheredge, "Transgenderism Two: Evidence and Identity".

parents whose child has fallen victim to an authoritarian social service, wielding power to "transition" a child.

Transitioning, then, is one of many euphemisms that refers to taking a person's healthy sexual organs and destroying what they actually have for the sake of what they can never have, which is the integral identity of the opposite sex. A boy or a girl cannot even have the "appearance" of the opposite sex, but ends up with a facsimile outcome which, in reality, is both irreversible and entails ongoing medical care. How is this not a variety of harms which arise out of the ideological grip of gender ideology?[2]

In general, then, the harm, is not neglible; nor, to be real, can the assessment of evidence be simplistic. After all, if a judge can assess the significance of a mother being dominated by gender ideology, to the point that she cannot consider an alternative response, nor can the clinician who was called on the mother's behalf assess alternative responses to the boy, then it is clear that this kind of evidence of ideological "capture" is real. As, in the end, it would be the mother who influenced the child's decision, along with the clinician, to the point that a twelve-year-old would scarcely understand what is happening and that, in fact, his health is about to be seriously compromised. Furthermore, the equally serious objection is that if the clinician cannot consider alternative treatments but, instead, uses a historical narrative to irrelevantly justify channelling a twelve-year-old into

[2] Cf. The Institute for Theological Encounter with Science and Technology, ITEST Webinar: https://www.youtube.com/watch?v=j_Nk3mwiyIQ.

transitioning, then a similar question should be asked about the professionalism of ideologically "captured" clinicians[3].

Similarly, why even now, has the National Health Service not complied with a request for data on this subject? As one journalist has put it:

> 'The first NHS study into 'early pubertal suppression in a carefully selected group of adolescents with gender identity disorders' began in 2011. The study yielded so little that, 15 years on, almost nothing meaningful has been learned.
>
> 9,000 young people have already been through the Gender Identity Development Service (Gids) and roughly 2,000 progressed to adult services. Knowing what happened to these children is vital'[4].

Let us remember, too, that the Cass Review criticised the gender clinics for their lack of record keeping. But, what is more, why did this lack of record keeping arise when, in reality, it is essential to good healthcare to monitor outcomes, especially in a controversial field of medicine where, in general, there are not good, promising results, to support what is called 'gender affirming care'? Moreover,

---

[3] Cf. Etheredge, *Transgenderism Two: Evidence and Identity*, a close reading of three documents, including that of Judge Strum's custody case of a twelve-year-old; it is now published: https://enroutebooksandmedia.com/ transgenderismtwo/.

[4] Lara Brown, 24th June, 2026, "Why is Baroness Cass backing another puberty blocker trial?": https://spectator.com/article/there-remains-insufficient-information-about-the-long-term-consequences-of-puberty-blocker-use-in-gender-questioning-children/.

as we will see below, there is a provision for what records there are to become publicly available:

> '[In the UK a] statutory instrument in question is a carve-out in the Gender Recognition Act that permits researchers investigating long-term outcomes to handle information relating to individuals with a Gender Recognition Certificate, something that would otherwise be unlawful.
>
> But no progress on linking patient data has been made. The Health Secretary, James Murray, was asked about the study on Tuesday and provided no timeline for when the NHS would deliver the information'[5].

In a word, there is a lamentable lack of cooperation, which the Cass Review had already found among gender clinics in the UK, even with respect to this ongoing request to contribute to a project about 'linking patient data'. Why is this?

***A variety of contributors which show, more widely, what contributes to this discussion on medical harm?***

Dr. Catherine Llewellyn, a psychiatrist, reflects on the harm that is being done to young people in the name of medically uncorroborated programs, and who is beginning to see the need for new Australian guidelines:

---

[5] Lara Brown, 24th June, 2026, "Why is Baroness Cass backing another puberty blocker trial?"

'Meaningful change to support the improved health of trans youth requires an uncompromising return to the highest standard of evidence-based medicine. But when we do, we will also need to brace ourselves for the harm that may have already been caused'[6].

Note what a more recent author says: 'The diagnostic criteria for gender dysphoria relies entirely on subjective self-reports and behavioural observations. There is no objective physical pathology'[7]. And what is very troubling too, 'the UK lacks a nationally recognised training programme for gender

---

[6] Catherine Llewellyn, "Does the gender-affirming model provide trans youth the healthcare they need? There are good reasons to think it doesn't": https://www.abc.net.au/religion/catherine-llewellyn-gender-affirming-healthcare-for-trans-youth/105319920. Dr. Catherine Llewellyn is a fellow of the Royal Australian and New Zealand College of Psychiatrists (FRANZCP) and completed advanced training in both Child and Adolescent Psychiatry and Addiction Psychiatry. She is also a fellow of the Australasian Society of Lifestyle Medicine (FASLM).' Cf. also, Hannah Barnes, May 27th, 2025, "Exclusive: Why Wes Streeting changed his mind on cross-sex hormones: The evidence that shifted the government's position on providing the treatment to children is revealed here":

https://www.newstatesman.com/politics/health/2025/05/exclusive-why-wes-streeting-changed-his-mind-on-cross-sex-hormones: 'It emerged last week (https://x.com/hannahsbee/status/1925153686994448830) that the Health Secretary was "actively reviewing" whether to restrict or ban the prescription of cross-sex hormones to children who want to transition to another gender …. The *New Statesman* can exclusively reveal the contents of the expert clinical reports which persuaded the government to change direction.' Thus, the increasing recognition of the irreversible harm brought about by puberty blockers and cross sex hormones proceeds apace.

[7] "Through the Looking Glass Through the Looking Glass: A SEEN in Publishing report into trans activism in children's literature and library services", Chapter 6: "The Medical Harms of 'Gender Affirmative Care' A Biology in Medicine GP, p. 66: https://www.transgendertrend.com/childrens-trans-themed-books/.

identity healthcare specialists'[8]. Indeed, 'according to the 'gender affirming model' the physical body can and should be altered, and the child's internal experiences cannot and should not be explored'[9].

Similarly, note the experience, research, and thinking through that a gynaecologist went through as she questioned more and more the removal of healthy wombs of young girls who appeared with no other motivation than that they did not want their womb. Dr. Karla Solheim went from relying on others to validate the claim that this was a constructive act to discovering that it had less and less authoritative research or accountability from those who advocated it.

She said: '*It is time to question whether "gender dysphoria" as an indication in and of itself for hysterectomy, without abnormal bleeding, pain, or any other diagnosis, should continue to bypass all of the checks and balances inherent in our healthcare system for major surgery.*

[8] "Through the Looking Glass", p. 67, a question I brought up in "Transgenderism: Evidence and Identity" (forthcoming from En Route Books and Media: https://enroutebooksandmedia.com/transgenderismtwo/. Cf. also the chapters on 'exceptionalism', which shows how the clinical use of hormones and surgery have circumvent the usual requirements for these procedures on minors or young people (Chapter 6); but, in addition, Chapter 7 shows how the "trans-self-identification" model of diagnosis completely disregards the psychological understanding of child development: "The Psychological Implications of Social and Medical Transition and the Gender Affirmation Approach", Dr Clea Thompson, D.Clin.Psych, M.A (Hons), Consultant Clinical Psychologist.

[9] "Through the Looking Glass", Chapter 7, p. 75.

*My fellow gynecologists, we are people of science. We know right from wrong. We care about our patients. We can find the courage to do this*[10].

Riittakerttu Kaltiala, a professor that pioneered gender-affirming care, started to notice that there were 'droves' of girls with gender dysphoria, that there was a proactive activist mentality among some "professionals" who were turning it into a human rights issue that young people had a right to this care and, as such, obscuring the question of whether hormones and surgery were an appropriate treatment. Kaltiala was already coming across de-transitioners and had reservations that these treatments were overlooking many who presented with psychiatric problems[11]. Now, then, Kaltiala has changed her methods and, while Finland has not banned 'puberty blockers, cross [sex] hormones and surgery' they are making progress with 'adopting new guidelines that insist on more holistic treatments that examine broader mental health challenges and sexuality issues faced by young patients'[12].

---

[10] Dr. Karla Solheim, MD, FACOG, May 27th, 2025, "It's Time for Liberal Physicians to Rethink American Gender Medicine: The Ethics of the Gender Affirming Hysterectomy": https://karlasolheim.substack.com/p/its-time-for-liberal-physicians-to.

[11] Riittakerttu Kaltiala, October 30th, 2023, 'Gender-Affirming Care Is Dangerous. I Know Because I Helped Pioneer It': https://www.thefp.com/p/ gender-affirming-care-dangerous-finland-doctor?r=e6yg3

[12] David Penberthy, August 15th, 2025, "'The situation has totally changed': Finnish expert to talk at Australian gender dysphoria conference": https://archive.is/20250815103833/https://www.theaustralian.com.au/nation/the-situation-has-totally-changed-finnish-expert-to-talk-at-australian-gender-dysphoria-conference/news-story/6fb4386b9872b24a82cebcbec7e17dc9#selection-639.0-639.101.

'Meanwhile, in Austria 4 minors underwent breast removal in 2011 but in 2023 that 'number … surged to 128'. Furthermore, politicians seem to be contemplating a law that would fine or imprison gender critical parents or clinicians who oppose the "transitioning" of children[13]. Talk about government overreach!'

In the words of a practicing psychiatrist: '*From 1995 to 2016, a period spanning over two decades and thousands of patient encounters, I did not meet a single transgender-identified young person. Today, I may encounter several transgender-identifying adolescents in a single afternoon clinic*'[14].

A social trend: 'there is a phenomenal relationship between the rise of social media, around 2010-2015, the coming of the pandemic and children being on-screen in a radically new immersion of influencers, and multiplication of disorientated young people. Thus the rate of Gender Clinic admissions or referrals went from a handful in the early days of the 1980s, to thousands upon thousands in more recent times. The change from outdoor to indoor play and the rise of unsupervised internet access and the spiked rising of

---

[13] Javier Villamor, June 17th, 2025, "Austria's Left Pushes for Jail Time For Those Opposing Trans Surgeries For Minors": https://europeanconservative.com/articles/news/austria-spo-liberals-greens-legislation-gag-law-protecting-minors-gender-reassignment/

[14] Dr. Kris Kaliebe, June 10th, 2025, "Society's Perfect Storm: Mental Health, Body Image, and Social Media: Dr Kris Kaliebe explores the intersection of online influence, self-image, and a growing mental health crisis": https://genspect.substack.com/p/societys-perfect-storm-mental-health

gender dysphoria, are not mere coincidences because the young, philosophically vulnerable age-group is particularly influenced by others'[15].[16]

'In a recent article a psychiatrist is both considering the "normality", as it were, of identity questioning youth and, at the same time, raising the possibility of the parent's involvement in the "virtual identity" of their child. On the one hand there has been an '8,000x increase of trans-identifying girls' which, in his view, is expressing a tendency for youth to identify in all sorts of counter-cultural ways, such as 'hippie, rocker, mod, punk, or goth' and parents[17], not without difficulty, would usually help to ground them in reality. But, on the other hand, what is different is that not only is there a 'social contagion', anti-discrimination law acting against professionals, or anybody questioning this contagion, there are also parents abdicating

---

[15] Francis Etheredge, "Transgenderism: A Question of Identity", En Route Books and Media, p. 336, in the prepublished manuscript:

[16] See also the number of "transitioners" who were using social media, or even children's computer programs, like Minecraft, but ended up being influenced by chats on gender ideology, cf. the chapter on personal experience, p. 52 particularly, in "Wolves in White Coates: How Doctors and Hospitals Pushed and Profited from the Fraud of "Gender Medicine"", 2026.

[17] Az Hakeem, Spring 2025, *Presser*, "Yes, Some Parents Are Overly Invested in Their Child Being the "Wrong Sex"": https://www.pressermag.com/spring-2025/yes-some-parents-are-overly-invested-in-their-child-being-the-wrong-sex. Az Hakeem, FRCPsych, MSc, is a consultant psychiatrist and group analyst. He is author of *DETRANS: When Transition Is Not the Solution.*

responsibility for helping their children and advancing the child's idea[18] of a virtual identity'[19].

***How did we get here?***

What seems to be a focus on what is happening to an increasing, growing, and disproportionately affected group of young girls, has a context which needs exploring: a context which is widespread, which includes pillorying dissent as phobic, anti-transgenderism, to the point of constituting a muzzle on legitimate discussion, disagreements, and treatment programs which opine non-invasive ways of helping these young people. However, just as a bruise is in the context of what happened, so there are reasons why this assault on young people is a part of a wider campaign to oppose the distinction between men and women, between male and female; and, therefore, this discussion is not just about the tragic effect of gender ideology on healthy young men and women, but on girls sports, men in women's toilets, men in women's changing rooms, and men in women's prison cells.

In other words, probably from *the Beijing conference on women in 1995* there has been a concerted program of influence, going back to earlier, radical feminist claims that required the abolition of the family and, going forward into innumerable, influential but non-binding agreements ever since. Indeed, if WPATH was founded in 1979, is there a connection between the founding of this

---

[18] Az Hakeem, Spring 2025, *Presser*, "Yes, Some Parents Are Overly Invested in Their Child Being the "Wrong Sex".

[19] Etheredge, "Transgenderism Two: Evidence and Identity".

organization and the radical elements that wanted to introduce 'gender' into the Beijing conference on women in 1995?[20] In other words, there has been a persistent, concerted, and wholesale campaign, emanating from the United Nations[21], and many other places, to destroy our understanding of sex, the family, and the natural nature of the human person. The Beijing declaration was a binding agreement which established that there are two sexes, male and female[22]. In truth, however, Beijing did not establish this biological truth; this biological truth was and is self-evident from the beginning (cf. Genesis, 1: 28); and, as such, permeates societies, either through the nature of marriage, in art, writings, and across the world. At the same time, just as science is beginning to understand the real difference that sex makes to the use of medicines, safety seats, and the compiling of statistics, so gender ideology dissembles a multitude of

---

[20] There is an excellent Webinar which introduces both the structure of the United Nations the Holy See and a specific work of watching, carefully, that words are not used in a way contrary to the good of real men and women. Jane Adolphe LLB/BCL/JCL/JCD (Professor of Law at Ave Maria School of Law, Founder & Executive Director of the International Catholic Jurists Forum) and John Klink, M.A. (Former Papal Diplomat and Chief Negotiator for the Holy See over UN World Summits in mid-1990s): 'Webinar on the UN and the Holy See', August 22nd, 2025: https://catholicsocialscientists.org/webinar-on-the-un-and-the-holy-see/.

[21] Cf. Francis Etheredge, October 25th, 2024, "We must fight gender ideology to preserve the concept of truth: There has been a systematic attempt to redefine language in a manner that makes contraception, abortion and now gender ideology more and more 'immersed' and 'implied' in non-binding agreements emanating from the United Nations bureaucracy": https://www.lifesitenews.com/opinion/we-must-fight-gender-ideology-to-preserve-the-concept-of-truth/.

[22] For the background research to this article, cf. Francis Etheredge, *Transgenderism: A Question of Identity*: https://enroutebooksandmedia.com/transgenderism/ and *Transgenderism Two: Evidence and Identity*, En Route Books and Media: https://enroutebooksandmedia.com/transgenderismtwo/.

modern developments to the detriment of women. On the other hand, as with Pope Francis' call for the reform of the United Nations[23], so the American's are calling for 'a UN that steers clear of controversial political issues and focuses on its core mission of peace and security.'[24]

In view of the natural tendency to form a world view, or a personal philosophy, which is generally characteristic of human beings, it follows that if critical thinking, the want of a good, metaphysical foundation, and a general ignorance of what is entailed in thinking through what is going on in ourselves or in society[25], then it follows that both parents and young people are particularly vulnerable to the insidious effects of multiple media platforms providing addictive but "loaded" content, skewing the understanding of people's perception of what is real[26]. Take, for example, a recent report on how gender

---

[23] Cf. Alessandro Gisotti, 25th December, 2015, "Pope Francis and the need for a more effective United Nations: In his speeches to the United Nations, as well as in "Fratelli tutti," Pope Francis has always encouraged a reform of the UN to give real concreteness to the concept of "a family of nations," at the same time urging greater efforts towards multilateralism": https://www.vaticannews.va/en/pope/news/2022-04/pope-francis-united-nations-war-ukraine.html.

[24] Stefano Gennarini, 2026, ""Woke" Muddies UN Secretary General Race": https://c-fam.org/friday_fax/woke-muddies-un-secretary-general-race/.

[25] Cf. *Faith and Reason*, 83 etc; but also *The Splendor of the Truth*, by St. John Paul II.

[26] Note the "datafication of reality" p. 17 of Christopher M. Reilly, May 2026, "AI and the Reduction of Truth: A Eucharistic Alternative": https://www.mdpi.com/2077-1444/17/5/551; and the impoverishment of relationships which arise out of undisciplined use media platforms (cf. Pope Leo XVI, "Magnificent Humanity", paragraphs 100, 139-141: https://www.vatican.va/content/leo-xiv/en/encyclicals/documents/20260515-magnifica-humanitas.html#Dependencies_and_societal_control.

ideology has been taken on by children's book publishers and, in effect, contributed to the creation of a cultural climate that induces children to think in terms of gender ideologists' claim, namely, that a person can be in the wrong body[27]. Thus, while even some Catholic authors thought gender dysphoria was independent of the cultural climate[28], there is now so much evidence of the presence of gender ideology in so many aspects of our social life that it is impossible to ignore the possibility that this was a long-term strategy. If 'the earliest books published for children following the 2015 Transgender Equality Inquiry, when the huge push to get transgender activism into schools really started.'[29], then it is likely that this was already a

---

[27] "Through the Looking Glass Through the Looking Glass", p. 7: 'Yet when SEEN in Publishing was commissioning chapters, the feeling was that gender affirmation has really got its claws into publishing staff, authors and librarians largely because there is a great deal of biological illiteracy in the literary world'. And, of course, children's literature is just one of many sources that seek to influence the induction of a gender ideology mentality in children and young people. As the doctor who has written chapter one of this book says: 'Teaching a child that gender can define sex and that the body should be changed to match this shifting idea is irresponsible and unethical' (p. 21).

[28] Cf. Transgender Health at the Intersection of Theology, Science, and Politics by Fr. Charles E. Bouchard, OP, PhD and Peter J. Smith, MD, MA, p. 4: Published in "First Principles", February 2025: https://faithscience.org/wp-content/uploads/2025/04/FiRST-Principles-February-2025-Vol-56-1.pdf. Gender dysphoria and gender incongruence are diagnosable conditions that are distinct from any gender ideology or cultural trend.' At the same time the authors present the option of hormones and surgery as if they are "neutral" treatments and not in and of themselves mutilation. Further, their distinction between physical sex and brain sex is based on an extrapolation of what happens in the case of an angel fish, which is discussed more fully in "Transgenderism Two: Evidence and Identity".

[29] Through the Looking Glass, p. 22.

watershed in a development which had precedents[30]. What is more, the books promote, to children, not what is your name but "What is your pronoun?" when they meet another child[31]. Indeed, the ideas in a pilloried author and a banned book were: 'simply that sex is biological and that gender is a social construct. What the activist teachers objected to was children being told the truth'.[32]

By contrast, Christianity's emphasis on both personal and corporate responsibility for what a person does and for what goes on in society, is itself a training in the real identity of individuals and society; but, on the contrary, in the world view of gender ideology there is a pervasive emphasis on non-personal groups in which people are reduced to labels and the perception of real people is impeded[33].

### *Let us consider the wide-angle lens*

In an excellent book, *God: The Science: The Evidence: The Dawn of a Revolution*[34], we can see that evidential science is not always well received. The science that recognized that it was possible that the universe was expanding, that this expansion pointed back to a beginning, and that the "anthropic conditions", as they are called, the

[30] "Through the Looking Glass": One advocacy organization was founded in 1997, p. 24.

[31] "Through the Looking Glass", p. 29.

[32] "Through the Looking Glass", p. 34.

[33] Gavin Ashenden, "He was Wounded not White. How the Good Samaritan would have saved Henry": https://www.youtube.com/watch?v=R83-vDneP5A.

[34] Originally written in French by Michel-Yves Bollore and Olivier Bonnassies, and many others, Translated into English, in 2025, by Rebecca M. West and Christine Elizabeth Jones, and published by Palomar editions, Luxembourg.

conditions that permit human life, are both extremely subtle and, at the same time, very precise, was rejected by both communist and nazi regimes. Thus, as many scientists have said, if the measurements of any number of variables were different, human life on earth would be impossible. The reception of these observations and conclusions was more than mixed; there was an especial hostility to them in communist Russia and in nazi Germany but, also, anywhere where there was a fear of introducing the possibility of a beginning and, therefore, of a creative act of God. The reason for this opposition was not scientific, it was that these modern findings contradicted the dominant world view, in these places, that entailed understanding 'reality within a strict materialist framework': 'reality exists in matter alone and not in any other dimension, least of all the "spiritual"'[35]. For, if it was conceded that the nature of the universe is evidence for God, then God exists; and, if God exists, then the implication is that human beings are not free to do what they like to one another: that there is, in reality, a transcendent source to human morality: a morality which calls us to do good and avoid evil (cf. *Veritatis Splendor*[36]).

What we see, then, is that this same reaction of rejecting a point of view which advocates acceptance of the basic duality of the sexes, as male and female, is at root an anti-life and anti-Christian world view. This rejection of the duality of sex, that man is male or female, has now led to a parallel academia as a number of the proponents of

---

[35] *God the Science The Evidence*, p. 130.

[36] St. John Paul II, *Veritatis Splendor*, paragraphs 38-64: https://www.vatican.va/content/john-paul-ii/en/encyclicals/documents/hf_jp-ii_enc_06081993_veritatis-splendor.html.

sex being binary have been driven out of employment, silenced, or accused of a transphobic behaviour when all they are doing is advocating a science-based biological approach that recognizes two sexes[37]. At the same time, a number of editors will not publish common terms like "man", "woman", "parent", "mother", "father" using clumsy terms which reduce women, particularly, to a kind of functional part of the body; one of the skewed requests was that ""women" [woman, adult female] be replaced with "people with female-identified reproductive organs""[38]. The irony of this is that even if a man has had surgery and had his sexual organ changed to "imitate" that of a woman, he is both a mutilated man and without 'female-identified reproductive organs'.

---

[37] Max Thompson, 9th of June, 2026, "Trans activism has turned Oxford into a toxic wasteland of censorship: The shutting down of Michael Foran's lectures proves that free speech is still in danger on campus": https://www.spiked-online.com/2026/06/09/trans-activism-has-turned-oxford-into-a-toxic-waste-land-of-censorship/; 'Foran [an Oxford academic] is far from alone. Last year, Professor Alice Sullivan (https://www.bbc.co.uk/ news/articles/cwyx3y84ln9o) – who had led a government commission recommending that data on biological sex and gender identity be recorded as distinct categories – endured a similar experience at the University of Bristol. In 2021, philosopher Kathleen Stock was hounded from her post at Sussex University because of her gender-critical views. And trans activists are more than happy to target students, too, as the cases of Connie Shaw and Thea Sewell depressingly demonstrate.' But there is the wider influence of this type of "targeting dissent" namely that of intimidating many ordinary people, whether professionals or not, from objecting to the radically destructive practices of gender ideology advocates.

[38] Karleen Gribble, 3rd March, 2026, "Erasing the Word "Woman": The desexing of language in women's health research and care is a story of the marginalisation of science, cultural imperialism, and abuse of power: https://quillette.com/2026/03/03/erasing-the-word-woman-trans-healthcare-mothers-breastfeeding/.

### ***Depersonalization: When a person is an objectified expression of an ideology***

A woman-person, just as a man-person, is an integral whole. This is because the woman's reproductive system is not an external "add on"; it is an integral system, which is endocrinal, ovulatory, and intimately integral to her whole body, including the nature of her hips, breasts, psychological awareness, all of which expresses the outcome of her XX chromosomes which, themselves, are integral to her whole genetic inheritance and development. Indeed, the whole problem of changing sex, whichever way the change goes, is not a change of sex but of an outward group of purely external, unintegrated, facsimiles. What these external changes say, as it were, is that a person is not a whole but some kind of chosen combination of bits; and, therefore, the person, which is the whole, is depersonalized. In other words, it is no longer a matter of a recognizable name and sex; but an unrecognizable combination of alterations, which, while being linguistic and to do with appearance, progress a "captured" person along a conveyor belt to more and more radically non-functional changes.

The discussion about a person confused about their sex is one thing. However, thinking that he or she is born in the wrong body, is an unfounded claim from the beginning; and, therefore, says more about the proponents of it, spreading confusion, than there really being a reality beyond that induced confusion. The exceptional cases which do occur, which are a biologically based intersex condition or a genuinely occurring psychological problem are, in principle, treatable. But, in the present discussion, "intersex", which is a genuine biological condition of the presence of both sexual organs, male and female, has been turned into a "middle sex", which it is not. Similarly, psychological disturbance, or trying out identities, which could be discussed, are often forbidden the talking types of treatment because of the claim that it is a retrograde conversion therapy: a therapy reminiscent of a type of forced rehabilitation of homosexual men. In other words, there is no discrimination as regards the variety of real types of human problems and, what is more, there is a "victim" narrative that makes any critical discussion of transgender ideology automatically toxic, phobic, and anti-transgenderist.

## PART IV

# SALVATION IS GOD'S RESCUING MISSION

In general, as we can see from the various reports that are emerging about gender ideology, there is an increasing wealth of evidence concerning its harm, the problematic thinking that it expresses without, usually, any self-critical reflection upon it, suggesting that there is more to what drives gender ideology than is commonly recognized. In other words, there is some kind of agenda at work if, as is often the case, there is a drive to suppress criticism, inhibit professionals from engaging in legitimate discussion of gender ideologists methods and a fear of legitimately different approaches to funnelling young people through a one response fits all, namely, that anyone must believe what the child says if he or she identifies with the opposite sex. For, as we know, children, young people, and indeed many others, can both be changeable and very influenced in what they are doing as their judgement and life experience may well be underdeveloped.

It is not sufficient, then, to draw upon the natural resources of reason and evidence; but, rather, to investigate both the roots of what leads to confusion about a person's identity and, at the same time, to recognize that there are many false trails in the course of fulfilling that ancient goal: "Know thyself". In what remains of this book, therefore, there are a number of reflections concerning the identity of the human person and the goal of human life. So, whatever the reasons that motivate gender ideologists there is a necessary wider reflection on what constitutes human identity; and, as such, these wider considerations are a valid contribution to the search that each one of us can undertake in answer to that dictum: "Know thyself".

To use an analogy, just as there are forces that can disintegrate an object as it is flung faster and faster in a circular motion, going nowhere, as it were, so there are forces that resist disintegration and indeed help to maintain the integrity of an object. But, to change the analogy, we need to come out of the "spin" and focus on the reality of who and what we are. And, as I have experienced myself, there is a help that goes beyond the harm that we have experienced: a help that comes from the word of God; and, indeed, therefore, from the power and creativity of God Himself.

***Discussion: Prophetic Church Documents***

The more I read and reread the documents of the *Second Vatican Council*, particularly *Gaudium et Spes*, (GS) the more I see that the Fathers of the Council were inspired to see that "once God is forgotten, the creature is lost sight of as well' (GS, 36). In other words, the world view, as it were, of gender ideology is a complete rejection of a Christian anthropology; it is probably inspired by an anti-population agenda as it specifically targets the possibility of young people growing up with a healthy sexuality, marrying, and having children.

By generating an identity crisis, gender ideologists are turning young people against their own bodies, and thus they achieve a nullification of these young people's God-given sexuality. By turning young people in on themselves, taking them out of social circulation, focusing them on bodily preoccupations which are, in effect, a rejection of their bodies, and insisting that these young people use made up words for what they are, there is a kind of viral narrative being introduced into their lives. This narrative tends to alienate them from their families, especially if their families disagree with the new language, such that gender ideology constitutes a rejection of the individual as a real person and the family as a real social reality. At the same time, having orchestrated a prejudicial use of the law, in some places it is possible for authoritarian social services to take a child into custody and promote, in effect, some kind of transitioning against the level-headed rejection of it by his or her parents. In the first place, then, gender ideology is anti-true individuality: an individuality which expresses the unique instance that each one of us is, whether male or female, a psychosomatic whole: either a man or a woman. In order to promote this, there is a false emphasis on the so-called claim that "sex" is determined at birth; however, biologically, a child's sex is determined at conception as, owing to two XX chromosomes a child is a girl or if there are XY chromosomes the child is a boy.

Thus, gender ideologists express an anti-family and an anti-God mentality. It is anti-family because the rest of the family of the "ideologically captured child" is now riven with conflicts concerning the support or contradiction of the child's new language especially, as it is often claimed, that the parents can either have a dead child or one that they agree can transition. And, to transition, as has already been said, is to become biologically incapable of fertility, having had genuine and integral body parts either corrupted by hormones or surgically destroyed, being replaced by infertile facsimiles. The reality of transition, then, is not from one sex to another, it is from the possibility of a healthy sexuality to a non-functioning sexuality: a sexuality that has been neutered and mutilated. All the while this is wrapped up in a legal and antagonistic rejection of contradiction: that to contradict this view is to express, not legitimate criticism, but a phobic and discriminatory rejection of transgender individuals. Gender ideology is, therefore, anti-God because God created man and woman 'to be fruitful, multiply, fill the earth and subdue it' (Gn. 1: 28).

According to gender ideologists, then, the body is not an integral expression of the human person, the whole of which is 'body and soul' (GS, 14); and, more deeply, the whole human person is not a gift to be received with gratitude. Rather, the material manifestation of the person is, precisely that, a kind of plastic flesh which can be manipulated and, in the process, loses its original, functioning integration as an expression of the whole person. A facsimile opening where once there was a male organ, or a facsimile male organ where once there was an opening, are no more integrated when it comes to the whole human being who has been mutilated, than makeup is integral to the person's face who is wearing it.

The Fathers of the *Second Vatican Council*, then, set out an anthropology, an account of the human person, which is not only true but is incredibly relevant for our times; for, in a certain way, it preempts precisely the disassociation of the "self" and the "body" which is so characteristic of gender ideology.

> 'Man, though made of body and soul, is a unity. Through his very bodily condition he sums up in himself the elements of the material world. Through him they are thus brought to their highest perfection and can raise their voice in praise

freely given to the creator. For this reason man may not despise his bodily life' (GS, 14).

### *Humanae Vitae: A perception of the loosening of the gift's value*

To put Pope St. Paul's VI document in perspective, we live in a time of multiple medical scandals. Beginning with the Nazis, there were atrocious experiments upon people in the extermination camps, along with the terrible slaughter of any number of human beings. Not to mention other slaughters in different parts of the world. With respect to the pill, there was already the process of manufacturing contraceptives, using ignorance and extremely high doses of hormones to the point of destroying women's health. Subsequently, putting women on contraceptives has become an endless money maker, upon which even ardent feminists remark[1]. At the same time, there was the Tuskegee scandal of antibiotics being withheld from black men so that a venereal disease could be studied[2].

---

[1] Shulamith Firestone, *The Dialectic of Sex: The Case for Feminist Revolution*, 1970; cf. my dialogue with her book in Etheredge, *Mary and Bioethics: An Exploration*: https://enroutebooksandmedia.com/maryandbioethics/; but also another author who wrote on her experience of being on contraceptives and how a pharmaceutical company responded to her complaints (discussed in Holly Grigg-Spall, *Sweetening the Pill*, 2013; cf. my discussion with her book in Etheredge, *Human Nature: Moral Norm*, 2023: https://enroutebooksand-media.com/humannature/; and cf. also, *The Word in Your Heart: Mary, Youth, and Mental Health*: https://enroutebooksandmedia.com/wordinyourheart/.

[2] Cf. Dr. Mary Ann Urlakis' "Foreword" to *The Human Person: A Bioethical Word*: https://enroutebooksandmedia.com/bioethicalword/. Cf. too, the careful evaluation of this medical abuse, that distinguishes the people responsible for this event from the place, 'Tuskegee', while nevertheless seeking to reflect on what actually happened through examining the historical record: Faith E. Fletcher, Sophie

Abortion, then, in its own way, contributes to this misuse of the natural order as it is literally destroying a human life, harming women, and encouraging a materialist mentality which "uses" the living, embryonic person as either disposable material or a "readymade" source for organ extraction. Thus, abortion is constantly denying that each human life-is-an-unmerited-gift. More widely, there is now death by organ stealing and unimpeded embryo experimentation. Have we all forgotten that each one of us was once, or still is, whether frozen or experimented upon, a gift: the gift of an embryonic human person?[3]

In 1968, not long after the closing of the *Second Vatican Council*, St. Paul VI brought out what has been one of the most controversial Vatican documents ever. Paul VI objected to an instrumentalization of sex: that sex can be divorced from the personal communication of husband and wife and that they can deliberately exclude the possibility of conceiving a child. Contraception, or being against conception, is different, in principle, from recognizing a need to space children, for good reason or reasons; and, as such, entails recognizing the natural rhythms of the woman's cycle and a willingness, on the part of both spouses, to accept and to enter into a collaborative

---

Schott, Virginia A. Brown, Nancy Berlinger and Stephen O. Sodeke, November 27th, 2023, "Newly Released Documents from Untreated Syphilis Study: Ethical, Just, and Respectful Use of Archival Materials": https://www.thehastingscenter.org/newly-released-documents-from-untreated-syphilis-study-ethical-just-and-respectful-use-of-archival-materials/ But then also see a more full-scale book on being open to life and its opposite called: *Human Nature: Moral Norm*: https://enroutebooksandmedia.com/humannature/.

[3] Cf. Etheredge, *The Salvation of the Embryonic Person: Beginning with the Incarnation and the Immaculate Conception*: https://enroutebooksandmedia.com/salvationofembryonicperson/.

mentality in the marriage. Contraception, however, which divorces sex and procreation, substituting lust or infatuation for love, is already a manipulation of the human body: as if the body does not express the person. The development of contraception caused immense suffering to the Puerto Rican women who were inadvertent guinea pigs with respect to this development; and, in general, reflects a tendency to commercialize the person and use them as a market for endless, unnecessary drug regimes, constituting a ready market for pharmaceutical companies. Separating sex and procreation is, already, like aborting an embryonic human being, a step and more than a step in the direction of gender ideology. This is because the whole human person is treated as if he, or she, whether as an adult or a child, are material to be manipulated, extinguished, or experimented upon.

Gender ideology, then, was given a beginning, as it were, in the atrocious and egregious attacks of what went before it in terms of contraception, abortion, and experimentation on human embryos and now, more and more, we see the same disregard for the meaning of the human person, suffering, and the difficulties of life, in the march towards euthanasia: the deliberate death of a human being. If there is no integral relationship between human personhood, and being male or female, then being male or female become "material expressions" of a choice: a choice that is imposed upon the human being and not one which arises out of his or her natural reality. What gender ideology develops, then, is the tendency to view the human being as a project of choice; but of choices that do not arise out of the whole person – but choices which are an imposition of the will upon a part of a person's natural identity.

On the other hand there is an erosion, as St. Paul VI would say, of marriage as 'the mutual gift of themselves' (*Humanae Vitae*, 8); and, as St. John Paul II went on to say, negatively, that contraception turns the reciprocal gift of husband and wife into a lie. In contraception, people take the "gift" from what is given in the act of giving and, consequently, do not open themselves to the whole gift of each giving themselves to the other. Being open to life, then, while not automatically bringing about the existence of a child, does not deny the possibility of becoming a mother or a father, exclusively, through each other. In other words, all these negative actions tend to distort, minimize, or undervalue the person-as-gift; and, if the person is no longer a gift, then what constitutes the person is no longer a "given".

### *The theology of the body: the person-as-gift*

What St. Paul VI and St. John Paul II articulated, then, was a theology of gift; and, as such, drew upon the mystery articulated in the *Second Vatican Council*:

> Jesus Christ 'has opened up new horizons closed to human reason by implying that there is a certain parallel between the union existing among the divine persons and the union of the sons of God in truth and love. It follows, then, that if man is the only creature on earth that God has wanted for its own sake, man can fully discover his true self only in a sincere giving of himself.' (GS, 24).

The gift of man, male or female, is a particular gift, resonating with the mystery of God Himself, in the mystery of that amazing gift of creation itself: that, from all eternity, God brought to exist what did not exist.

Gender ideology, then, specially targets the reality of each human life being a gift: that the gift is total and all inclusive: that each one of us is a psychosomatic whole: a bodily-person-gift: male or female. This is because gender ideology turns the "externality" of that gift against the natural "internality" of that gift. In other words, on the one hand there is a rejection of the endless permutations of being a male or a female individual person and, on the other hand, there is a rejection of the integral gift of human personhood, in itself, as male or female. Thus there is a rejection of our personal reality-as-gift; and, if there is a rejection of our personal reality-as-gift, there is a rejection of the giver: of God. What we have, then, in the world view of gender ideology, is a rejection of God and human reality which parallels that of the communist and nazi authorities' rejection of the new discoveries in mathematics and physics - - precisely because to accept them was to open the door to the possibility of the existence of a finite creation and the reality of creation as a witness to the existence of God-as-Creator.

In rejecting the bodily expressed personhood of being male or female, there is a rejection of the integral anthropology of the Christian vision; and, therefore, there is a rejection, not only of the integral nature of human personhood, one in body and soul, but of the vocation to which each of us is called: a vocation to love and service: both to each other and to God. There is now no subordination of created reality to a Creator; and, as *Gaudium et Spes* teaches: 'once God is forgotten, the creature is lost sight of as well' (GS, 36). And, if the creature is 'lost sight of as well' then so is the whole understanding of the origin of our imperfections through an original sin of disobedience and its impact on our ability to understand ourselves and to live the truth in love. Gender ideology replaces sin, and human imperfection, with a human recipe of mutilation: that there is no significance to the reality of being "given" to be male or female; rather, just as our existence seems to be an expression, for some, of 'being in the wrong body', so we can do what we like to the 'wrong body' to rectify it. Moreover, gender ideology develops a narrative of "injustice" to the point that anyone who objects gender ideology is automatically, and uncritically, guilty of perpetuating an injustice against people who claim to be in the "wrong body." The principle of "gift" is completely replaced by the imposition of the falsification of the integral unity of the human person: the falsification of the integral unity of the human person is a human inversion of the gift of human personhood: we become, tragically, the "self-made man", who no longer knows his or her reality in the light of being given the gift of human personhood.

> 'Man, though made of body and soul, is a unity. Through his very bodily condition he sums up in himself the elements of the material world. Through him they are thus brought to their highest perfection and can raise their voice in praise freely given to the creator. For this reason man may not despise his bodily life. Rather he is obliged to regard his body as good and to hold it in honor since God has created it and will raise it up on the last day. Nevertheless man has been wounded by sin. He finds by experience that his body is in revolt. His very dignity therefore requires that he should

glorify God in his body, and not allow it to serve the evil inclinations of his heart' GS, 14).

### *In conclusion*

'In reality it is only in the mystery of the Word made flesh that the mystery of man truly becomes clear' (*Gaudium et Spes*, GS, 22).

If there is a single answer to the good that God is seeking to bring out of this crisis concerning the truth that biological sex exists, it is that truth exists and that we are called to pursue it, even when it seems unlikely to be successful. For, given the tendency of human beings to distort human perception, it is both salutary and necessary to keep that particular door open: the search for truth in all its varied richness. However, as we can see from the testimonies of those who were led to question what they were doing, both because of their own experience of the surgical removal of healthy wombs, and that of the psychiatrist who noticed a dramatic increase in the number of young women coming through her clinic, there is hope that there is a new way forward from those who are open to the truth embodied in evidence. However, for those whose investment in gender ideology is ideological, whether because of money, anti-Christian views, anti-population policies, or for whatever reason, there is the power of litigation. Increasingly, then, de-transitioners, that is men or women who are reclaiming their original sex from conception, are filing lawsuits against those who "funnelled" them from obscure pronouns to wound-generating surgeries.

What emerges from all this is that what happens in a society which has lost its way, both philosophically and theologically, is that as the Christian worldview diminishes, is withdrawn, is criticised, and "objectified" as anti-progressive, both individuals and institutions are vulnerable to whatever the prevailing activists promote. For we are already immersed in a culture that overwhelms almost all of us with information without understanding, with bits but without the whole picture, with assertions rather than arguments, with the uncritical rather than the critical assimilation of what is proposed and, in addition, with a social antagonism to disagreement which makes it more and more difficult for people to object unless, very concretely, they are willing to lose their jobs, or to be persecuted. Moreover, the clearer it becomes that advocating for the existence of biological sex becomes an automatic exclusion from the pages of journals, not to mention public speaking forums, the more obvious it becomes that the alternative is to become part of another system of publishing and advocacy for biological sex as an enduring reality. Furthermore, there is the growing and widespread disparagement of actual science, genuine medical records, and the reality of verifiable evidence that pertains to what is cumulatively known, not just because it is historically consistent, but because it expresses the enduring continuity of truth with reality "as it is". At the same time, there are those who continue to promote the re-opening of the "space" for public debates as against the negative tendency not to argue, not to produce evidence, but to lambast, name-call, and persecute those who legitimately disagree with ideological claims. In other words, the law needs to explicitly, boldly, and simply distinguish legitimate differences of opinion and evidence from bald claims of discrimination and the toxification of disagreements.

What also emerges from all this is that there is a reality to the prophetic nature of Christian documents, especially those promulgated by the Magisterium of the Church, whether by Council or Papal document, such that they contribute very concretely to the formation of the worldview, the conscience, and the resources available to people generally. Together, then, these documents contribute, with the Scriptures, to raise our hope in the possibility of a power beyond ourselves, to free us from our 'hidden faults' (Psalm 19: 12). Indeed, 'so that the active potency of the faith be revealed again'[4]. And, more than that, that these instruments of the healing help of the Lord can lead to the hope that our hearts can be opened to the truth, to God and to each other. Furthermore, these developments are not without precedent; therefore, it is always valuable to cultivate our familiarity with the Tradition of the Church, which progresses with the help of the Holy Spirit (*Dei Verbum*, 8).

What finally emerges is that we need all the help we can receive when the culture we are immersed in rejects the whole principle of "reception": that we are the beneficiaries of the gifts of God. Thus, Mary and the Church, who express this principle of "reception", both personally and institutionally, are there to accompany us as we strive

---

[4] From Peter Seewald's "Foreword" to the book on Pope Benedict XVI'th called *Last Testament: I his own words*, translated by Jacob Phillips, London, New York, Bloomsbury, 2016, p. xiii; indeed, given the title of the book, it is ironic that this particular expression of Pope Benedict's thought is actually expressed by Peter Seewald. Nevertheless, Peter's expression is very apt as Pope Benedict wrote *Verbum Domini*, building on *Dei Verbum* of the *Second Vatican Council* and many other works.

to see and to act on the truth which really, objectively exists, particularly the truth that we are more than matter, that matter itself cannot think and that, therefore, we are different from purely inorganic, or even organic matter. And that recognizing this difference, that we are embodied, psychosocial beings, opens up the whole possibility of our being made in the image and likeness of the Blessed Trinity, which makes us, in reality, created from relationship, for relationship, through relationship. In other words, God invites us to constantly deepen our understanding of who we are, just as our society seems to lose the ground which had been gained, philosophically and theologically, that we may not only recover what is lost but become equipped, too, to answer the new "things" of the times in which we live. Perhaps, among these "new things", is a rediscovery of the power of the word of God to form our hearts in such a way that we will be more and more capable, like Christ Himself, of speaking "heart to heart": of being enlightened about our own reality, both individually and socially, and the reality of God.

Christ offers us a completing identity, an identity to be found in Him (*Gaudium et Spes*, 22), which does not distort but becomes who we are and opens upon the horizon of the history of salvation: a horizon which opens upon the mystery of man and the mystery of God and, at the same time, draws us into an ongoing illumination of our culture as we grasp, increasingly, the significance of what is going on[5].

---

[5] Cf. "Final Statement of the Workshop on Digital Rerum Novarum: Artificial Intelligence, Peace, Social Justice and Integral Human Development": https://www.pass.va/en/events/2025/digital_rerum_novarum/final_statement.html.

## PART V

# DO WE NEED "ANOTHER" PUBERTY-BLOCKER TRIAL?[1]

'The modified protocol [for a UK puberty-blocker trial] includes strengthened safeguards including the introduction of minimum ages of entry to the trial and more clearly defined discontinuation measures around safety for bone health, cognition, and vaginal bleeding as well as more detailed information for participants on fertility preservation'[2].

The organizers of the puberty blocker trial are proposing that the minimum age of entry is that of 11-year-old girls and 12-year-old boys, with parental consent[3].

It aims to provide evidence on how the timing of treatment affects quality of life, mental health, physical development, cognitive function, and gender-related distress'[4].

---

[1] Alison Holt, June 19th, 2026, "Minimum age of 11 set for UK puberty blocker trial": https://www.bbc.co.uk/news/articles/c892p2qdjjxo.

[2] "Update on the PATHWAYS clinical trial: As with all clinical trials, the MHRA's top priority is the safety and wellbeing of the trial participants": https://www.gov.uk/government/news/update-on-the-pathways-clinical-trial.

[3] Alison Holt, June 19th, 2026, "Minimum age of 11 set for UK puberty blocker trial".

[4] "Update on the PATHWAYS clinical trial".

***Discussion: What can a trial add to what is already known?***

The trial planners, then, already expect a number of possible harms in view of applying puberty blockers. The vaginal bleeding referred to is when the wall of the vagina is thinned[5] and can lead to bleeding, but it can atrophy too, owing to what is known to have happened to East German sportswomen[6]. Both are irreversible. Thus, there is already information available on the effect of administering these hormones.

What does 'fertility preservation' mean? Is that the same as preserving boys' sperm and girls' eggs? And, if so, how are they going to be obtained? This is precisely what a child does not understand and which de-transitioners discover later, when they want to conceive their own children and cannot if, that is, they have been subjected to puberty blockers, cross sex hormones and or surgery which are, in effect, atrophying or mutilating healthy sexual organs to produce facsimiles of the opposite sex.

---

[5] "Through the Looking Glass Through the Looking Glass: A SEEN in Publishing report into trans activism in children's literature and library services", Chapter 1: "What is Sex? Dr. Alice Hodkinson MA MBBS MRCGP MA Medical Ethics and Law", p. 17: 'Testosterone in women … can cause … an initial surge of sense of well-being and increased libido, but it often goes on to cause anxiety. It also causes atrophy or thinning to the genital tract which can be irreversible': https://www.transgendertrend.com/childrens-trans-themed-books/.

[6] Paul Steger, May 26th, 2025, "Doped then, transitioned now: The East German doping scandal is a tragic blueprint for the health effects of testosterone on female bodies. If known more widely, it could help both detransitioned and trans-identified women": https://genderstats.substack.com/p/doped-then-transitioned-now.

Where, furthermore, is the prior, talk-therapy option? What about parents who are convinced, ideologically, that their child is the opposite to his or her natural sex? What if 'the earliest books published for children following the 2015 Transgender Equality Inquiry, when the huge push to get transgender activism into schools really started'[7], are now producing the children and parents likely to be already disposed to "welcome" what is clearly a high-risk and unnecessary procedure? Where is objective parental and clinical advice to the found?

Are not these gender experimentalists not skewing the child's prospects of normal psychological and physical development for the sake of their own claims? This was precisely the question raised by Judge Strum, in Australia, whereby a mother wanted to "transition" her twelve-year-old son; and, for good reason, the judge forbade the custody of the child to go to the mother in view of the child being too young to understand what is happening, and the mother being so convinced of gender ideology as to be incapable of considering other options. At the same time, the advocacy for "transitioning" the child was based, not on evidence, but on the narrative that the so-called transgender group of people are a part of a historic process of victimization. None of which, as the judge rightly opined, had an immediate bearing on the custody of the child[8]. But, to those who need to know, this is

---

[7] "Through the Looking Glass", Chapter 2: "Trans-themed Children's Books: Stephanie Davies-Arai, Founder and Director, Transgender Trend, p. 22.

[8] Cf. The very detailed discussion of Judge Strum's judgement in "Transgenderism Two: Evidence and Identity", forthcoming from En Route Books and Media: https://enroutebooksandmedia.com/transgenderismtwo/;

precisely part of the manipulative strategy which includes threatening dissenters with slogans, like "transphobic", or with litigation via anti-discrimination laws, or with the following, generalised claim: "Do you want a dead son or a live daughter?". In other words, no discussion of the pros and cons of actual treatments, their methodology, and philosophy. Indeed, recently, a nurse of some forty years' experience, wrote an article reviewing the data on transgenderism and suicide and concluded:

> 'The article summarised six long-term historical studies produced in the Netherlands, Sweden, the United Kingdom, Denmark and Finland, which, like the Cass review in 2024, do not support the claims of the World Professional Association for Transgender Health about the increased risk of suicide'. Similarly, then, this article was pulled from the journal and the author was accused of 'negativity and hatred' for summarising '30 or 40 years worth of data'[9]. In other words, the author simply

---

but see also two prior books from which this one emerged. Transgenderism: A Question of Identity, published by En Route Books and Media: https://enroutebooksandmedia.com/transgenderism/. But also this subject began to emerge in Mary and Bioethics: An Exploration: https://enroutebooksandmedia.com/maryandbioethics/. Thus these books have been exploring the emergence of a type of radically destructive feminism which seeks to destroy the family, is anti-population, and already in the 1995 Beijing Conference on women, sought to introduce "gender" terminology – but it was rejected in favour of a biological definition of man and woman.

[9] Stephen Rice, July 15th, 2026, "Nurses' journal pulls suicide study over 'trans distress': Australia's biggest nurses union retracted a journal article on transgender suicide research and accused its author of 'hatred'. Now he's threatening to sue": https://archive.md/21CM1#selection-781.0-785.157.

objected to the narrative that there is a higher risk of suicide if "gender affirming care" is not pursued – from changing pronouns and clothes to hormones and surgery. In other words, the issue here, as in many other places, is the right to publish a well-founded article which is critical of "gender affirming care" claims.

Furthermore, then, there is the danger that a "puberty-blocker" trial puts children at risk of harm for the sake of what seems to amount to a "face-saving" exercise for a medical procedure that is generally discredited, in view of its actual harm to the young people who go through with it. Double mastectomy scars, changing an outward male organ into a facsimile of a female organ and vice versa, are actual harms in their own right. The Cass report already said that pronoun change is already putting a child on a path to life-changing procedures. Are these young people, then, already on that path, owing to all the propaganda that claims it is possible "to be in the wrong body"? A propaganda campaign which did not address the harms of these procedures, very often called them reversible[10] when they are

---

[10] This being one of the claims that allow those who regret these transitions to sue those who put them forward for these procedures, Ashley Bateman, July 9th, 2026, "Disfigured Texas Woman Allowed To Sue Therapist For Transgender Medicine Fraud": https://thefederalist.com/2026/07/09/ disfigured-texas-woman-allowed-to-sue-therapist-for-transgender-medicine-fraud/; and cf. the new legislation that may make help de-transitioners to claim for the remedial treatments they will need, Ashley Bateman, August 3rd, 2026, "Bill Would Make Insurance Cover Body-Acceptance Treatments For Trans Desisters": https://thefederalist.com/2026/08/03/bill-would-make-insurance-cover-body-acceptance-treatments-for-trans-desisters/

not, and has long been promoting itself in children's literature, schools and universities.

What about the clinics who never kept records on the several thousand who have been through their processes already? So, is a puberty-blocker trial a way of avoiding liability for what has happened already? Thus, it can be claimed, "we" are awaiting the outcome of a "properly" conducted trial before any litigation can proceed.

More widely again, in yet another international development, the Italian guide to gender affirming care said that it was,

> 'An affirmation-only guide, which offers a case study of social transition for a three-year- old Italian boy and advises paediatricians to refer teenagers to gender clinics "without judging" their requests, has had an unexpected effect.' The effect, as we shall see, is that of galvanizing opposition to this 'gender-affirming-care' document.
>
> In addition, this document gives 'the case study of "Liam", a 15-year-old girl who binds her chest, [and] the paediatrician stresses the importance of the mother "accepting her son's identity" and offers her information about "multidisciplinary care at specialist centres dedicated to gender incongruence", namely gender clinics[11].

[11] A woman who once worked in a gender clinic witnessed the 'lie', as she calls it, of 'gender-affirming-care': a lie that is layered and becomes more and more difficult to undo. In other words there is a time to say no, helpfully, and that time is at the first encounter with the lie. cf. LGB Courage Coalition and Jamie Reed, August 18th, 2026, "The same world that affirmed Jason

> The father, who does not go along with his daughter's male role, is blamed for "contributing to a conflictual family atmosphere'"[12]
>
> Again, there is a want of discrimination here in that working through conflict is an integral part of a parent-child relationship; and, in this case, it is especially significant that the father has seen the potential damage to his daughter and rightly objects to it. This is a healthy response to ideas which lead to real harm to children.

This document has, additionally, given the following advice: In "An introduction to the guide[13] [it] says: "Expressions such as 'It's just a phase', 'You're too young to know' or 'You'll see, it'll pass' … risk conveying a sense of devaluation or inadequacy at a stage of development when being listened to and feeling trusted

---

Arday affirmed my child as trans": https://lgbcouragecoalition.substack.com/p/the-same-world-that-affirmed-jason?r=2ij6zg.

[12] Bernard Lane, July 30th, 2026, "Blowback: An activist guide for paediatricians in Italy has, for the first time, roused many clinicians from silence and galvanised them into open opposition to the affirmative treatment model": https://www.genderclinicnews.com/p/blowback-697?r=130uly&triedRedirect=true.

[13] The guide is 'issued by the Italian Paediatric Society and the Cultural Association of Paediatricians under the title Beyond the Gaze: A Practical Guide to Gender Variance, Sexual Orientations and Same-Sex Parenting for a Welcoming Paediatric Clinic—have felt the need to publish a Q&A "technical document" in response to the critique of the petition': https://www.genderclinicnews.com/p/blowback-697?r=130uly&triedRedirect=true.

are fundamental.'"[14] In other words, the writers of the document cannot distinguish between advice which targets serious errors in self-understanding, and advice that seeks to devalue or deem a person as inadequate. These are distinct and separate problems. Advice can address false ideas, while affirming the person, precisely by distinguishing the trajectory of growing up from errors which can, and often are, a part of that process. Otherwise, it seems, the argument is that almost any and every idea a young person has about themselves has to be uncritically affirmed.

The unexpected effect of this Italian document is that many people who have been silent are now vocal in opposing this guide, whether as professionals or as parents[15]. In view, then, of how this Italian document portrays those who object to gender ideology, it clearly raises the concern, yet again, that those too close to gender ideology cannot see the harm it is doing to individuals, family relationships, and professional associations or practitioners who are critical of it. In view, then, of these objections to the unprecedented blanket acceptance of children and young people's erroneous claims, we can see that this is a timely reminder that there is not unanimity with respect to "gender-affirming-care" and that, therefore, this is a reason to take note of it being imprudent to pursue it further.

---

[14] Bernard Lane, July 30th, 2026, "Blowback: An activist guide for paediatricians in Italy has, for the first time, roused many clinicians from silence and galvanised them into open opposition to the affirmative treatment model".

[15] Bernard Lane, July 30th, 2026, "Blowback: An activist guide for paediatricians in Italy has, for the first time, roused many clinicians from silence and galvanised them into open opposition to the affirmative treatment model".

More widely, as scandals continue to surface concerning the negligent lack of psychological assessments of children eligible for so-called gender-affirming care[16], we get the impression that this lack of psychological assessment echoes WPATH's tendency to characterise such interventions as bordering on 'conversion therapy'. At the same time, although WPATH noted a possible element of coercion in the UK puberty-blocker trial, it does not actually object to this treatment program and laments that the cohort that will not receive it are being delayed reception of them; and, therefore, there is the implicit view that puberty-blockers are good for children. Clearly there is a group that will go ahead with puberty blockers and a group that do not. Thus, anonymously, WPATH says:

> 'Furthermore, as currently designed, the study may risk harm to those in need of treatment by delaying care for half of participating adolescents and by initiating puberty blockers later in adolescence when the balance of benefits and risks is less clear.'[17]

---

[16] Brad Crouch, August 16th, 2026, "SA Health review into WCH gender treatment of 22 children will be kept secret: Children received gender-affirming treatment at the WCH in breach of government guidelines - now SA Health wants to keep the probe into the scandal a secret": https://archive.md/oadBK#selection-779.0-783.157.

[17] January 8th, 2026, "For Immediate Release: WPATH and USPATH Join EPATH in Raising Ethical Concerns Over the UK Government's PATHWAYS Trial": https://wpath.org/wp-content/uploads/2026/01/Final-WPATH_EPATH-PATHWAYS-Holding-Statement.pdf.

Let us not forget that the UK children's study is advocating puberty-blockers for 11–12-year-olds; and, in principle, WPATH, does not object to this.

### *A Second Conclusion*

What is the possibility, then, that a target group of 11–12-year-olds is anything but "programmed" to think that they are in the "wrong body" without any objective, diagnosable evidence, without any counselling to help them? What about parental consent? Also, as in the case of Judge Strum's analysis, what if the parent is so convinced of gender ideology that they are incapable of discerning, critically, what is good for their child? In other words, if the parent cannot evaluate what the options are, either because they do not know them, or because they have already been convinced that puberty blockers are the only option, then they are not in a position to give valid consent. Thus, both child and parent, are not good candidates for informed consent. Thirdly, if there is already evidence of the harm of puberty blockers, cross-sex hormones and surgery that renders children and young people disfigured, then why is a so-called trial really necessary? If, then, the trial clinicians are not capable of assessing the evidence to date, of considering alternative strategies, as there has been no mention of counselling, then what hope is there for this being a valid and useful trial?

Furthermore, the irony in all this is that the legislation to prevent 'abusive conversion practices' can be applied to those who advocate gender ideology; for, from an almost non-existent problem there is now an all but overwhelming pro-gender ideology cultural environment[18]. So, can this legislation, which seems to pick up and hook into the narrative about injustice to those who have suffered 'abusive conversion practices' be considered an impartial plea for what needs to be done "today"? Indeed, if this legislation is passed, can it be used by de-transitioners to frame what it is like to being funnelled through from pronouns to devasting surgery?[19]

> In a new report, already quoted in this book, the introduction to the chapter on personal experience reads: 'These accounts—some by detransitioners and others by patients or the parents of patients who resisted the pressure to pursue sex-rejecting procedures—shed further light on the degree to which activists and providers have tried to force children to undergo potentially life-altering interventions.'[20]

---

[18] Office for Equality and Opportunity and Olivia Bailey MP , 26th June, 2026, "Government pushes forward with conversion practices ban to protect LGBT+ people from abuse: The government is banning abusive conversion practices in England and Wales to protect LGBT+ people from physical and psychological harm": https://www.gov.uk/government/news/government-pushes-forward-with-conversion-practices-ban-to-protect-lgbt-people-from-abuse

[19] Cf. Note the prevalence of manipulation and coercion in the reported experience of a number of detransitioners: "Wolves in White Coats": https://www.youtube.com/watch?v=OjuFx9Pd_Vo.

[20] P. 45 of "Wolves in White Coates: How Doctors and Hospitals Pushed and Profited from the Fraud of "Gender Medicine"", 2026.

Ultimately, then, WPATH has practiced, discussed, and logged many real changes to many people; and, therefore, it could be argued that WPATH needs to make all of their findings available for public scrutiny. The availability of WPATH's own internal experience and dialogue may well answer many if not all questions concerning what has been done in the name of 'gender-affirming-care'; and therefore, the question needs to be raised: Can WPATH be compelled to share what has been logged in private discussions - both for the sake of stopping what is harmful and helping to heal what has been done. Thus, as well, would this not diminish, if not abolish, the need for any further puberty hormone trials and what follows?[21]

### *A Third Conclusion*

Whether we are talking about gender ideologists, children, young people, those who are older, we are always talking about people who are greater, to paraphrase an expression of Pope Francis': we are always talking about people who are greater,

---

[21] Cf. Megan Block, July 29th, 2026, "Inside WPATH: Trans Surgeon Admits Patients May Experience Painful Complications": "Just because someone does not wish to maintain their vagina because of pain and discharge, jumping to regret should not be our first response": https://www.dailywire.com/news/trans-surgeon-admits-some-patients-may-not-maintain-their-vagina-due-to-brutal-complications; and cf. also Megan Brock, July 30th, 2026, "Inside WPATH: Trans Org Admits Need For Detransitioner Protocols While Pushing Child Sex-Changes": "There is a critical and undeniable need for detransitioner protocols — a reality acknowledged even by WPATH's own members": https://www.dailywire.com/news/wpath-files-trans-org-admits-need-for-detransitioner-protocols-while-pushing-child-sex-changes.

more complex, deeper, and more varied in their actual histories than any kind of stereotypical portrait of a person. Thus we both hope and pray that it is possible to engage others through evidence, through philosophy, through theology, in the course of their thinking through their understanding of what life is about. Let dialogue prevail; but, also, let prevention be the context of letting dialogue prevail.

# POSTSCRIPT

# EVIDENCE OR A SMOKE SCREEN

In general, 'The Federal Trade Commission ("FTC")' .... [claims it] 'has authority to regulate "deceptive" statements that mislead consumers'; and, in this instance, the FTC claims that it is the World Professional Association for Transgender Health (WPATH) which is misleading customers with deceptive statements. WPATH replies, denying it has misled, duped, or acted as if it is marketing a product or a service[1]. Thus, WPATH claims that it is not liable in that its medical opinions are 'non-actionable opinions about subjects on which there is "medical and scientific uncertainty."'[2] Reading through the presentation of WPATH's defence, it is possible to take the view that its statement is an overwhelming "wall" of citations, whether from journals or legal cases.

---

[1] UNITED STATES DISTRICT COURT FOR THE NORTHERN DISTRICT OF TEXAS FORT WORTH DIVISION. FEDERAL TRADE COMMISSION, et al., Plaintiffs, v. WORLD PROFESSIONAL ASSOCIATION FOR TRANSGENDER HEALTH, INC., a Texas corporation, et al., Defendants. Case No. 4:26-cv-00748-O

DEFENDANT WORLD PROFESSIONAL ASSOCIATION FOR TRANSGENDER HEALTH, INC.'S MEMORANDUM IN SUPPORT OF ITS MOTION TO DISMIS, p. 1; https://segm.org/sites/default/files/2026-08/WPATH %20Motion%20to%20dismiss_Aug%202026.pdf.

[2] Case No. 4:26-cv-00748-O. DEFENDANT WORLD PROFESSIONAL ASSOCIATION FOR TRANSGENDER HEALTH, INC.'S MEMORANDUM IN SUPPORT OF ITS MOTION TO DISMIS, p. 1.

Ultimately, does WPATH's claim to the right of 'free speech'[3], on the basis of which it publishes its views, override the actual, iatrogenic harm, or wounds, caused by practices advocated by them? Let us recall, an iatrogenic harm can both be an actual wound, among other things, and it can "include mental suffering via medical beliefs or a practitioner's statements.'[4] And, as the literature on detransitioners develops, many of the experiences of parents and their children include 'mental suffering' induced by such claims as "Do you want a dead daughter or a live son?": 'At her first appointment—approximately one hour long—clinicians told her parents she was "100% trans" and at high risk of suicide if not affirmed. Breen was only 12.'[5] The physical sufferings of so-called transitioners have been written about throughout this and previous books.

### *The Questionable Validity of Citations*

'The current version of those Standards of Care ("SOC-8"[6]) [published by WPATH] has a sixty-nine-page bibliography citing

[3] Cf. references to this right cited in this document: Case No. 4:26-cv-00748-O. DEFENDANT WORLD PROFESSIONAL ASSOCIATION FOR TRANSGENDER HEALTH, INC.'S MEMORANDUM IN SUPPORT OF ITS MOTION TO DISMIS, pp. 31-32, 35.

[4] "Iatrogenesis": https://en.wikipedia.org/wiki/Iatrogenesis.

[5] P. 45, and also p. 49, 51 of "Wolves in White Coates: How Doctors and Hospitals Pushed and Profited from the Fraud of "Gender Medicine"", 2026.

[6] E. Coleman, A. E. Radix, W. P. Bouman, et al. (2022) Standards of Care for the Health of Transgender and Gender Diverse People, Version 8, International Journal of Transgender Health, 23:sup1, S1-S259, DOI: https://www.tandfonline.com/doi/pdf/10.1080/26895269.2022.2100644.

over 1,500 scientific studies to support its guidance.'[7] As regards legal cases, whatever the merits of those quoted in WPATH's submission, there are many documented instances of legislation and the law being used to silence gender critical voices, whether in academia or in the public domain[8]. As regards journals and editing, it does not follow that a 'sixty-nine-page bibliography' in support of WPATH's claims constitutes anything other than coordinated support; in the experience of some writers, there is an editorial rejection of gender-critical writing.

> The author, Karleen Gribble, of the article from which these statements have been drawn, has traced the increasing frequency with which 'those working in maternal and child health have experienced pressure to avoid these terms [women, mothers] and desex our language.' Thus, biological sex has been increasingly removed from the vocabulary; and so, she says, 'since 2010, there has been a sharp increase in

---

[7] Case No. 4:26-cv-00748-O. DEFENDANT WORLD PROFESSIONAL ASSOCIATION FOR TRANSGENDER HEALTH, INC.'S MEMORANDUM IN SUPPORT OF ITS MOTION TO DISMIS, p. 1.

[8] Cf. the assorted cases in this and the previous two books. But, in addition, there are two more examples of the law being used to punish recognizing a man as a man although, in the second case, the argument was that calling a man a man was a form of 'the "intentional and pejorative use of the gender opposite… [to a] self-declared identity." How you prove an 'intentional and pejorative use' of a word is a moot point. Either way, there are many exchanges between people which, if all were taken to court, the court would be unworkable. Anna Slatz, August 14th, 2026, "Brazilian University Worker Convicted Of Criminal Transphobia, Sentenced To ONE YEAR In Prison For "Misgendering" Transgender Student": https://reduxx.info/brazilian-university-worker-convicted-of-criminal-transphobia-sentenced-to-one-year-in-prison-for-misgendering-transgender-student/.

the frequency of "assigned sex" and "sex assigned at birth," reflecting the new use of these phrases to supplant "biological sex" or simply "sex." On the one hand this use of language was 'to avoid distress and protect those people who call themselves transgender' and whom they see as vulnerable. On the other hand, 'Other individuals and organisations appear to have a broader intent to marginalise sex and to replace it with gender identity across the board, including in policy and data collection. Of course, to do this, it is necessary to obscure sex in language.' And so we see not only a marked increase in sexless language, such as 'pregnant person', 'chestfeeding', 'menstrators', but also its impact on journal submissions and editors. Thus it 'became clear that the desexing of all communications was the end goal' with a rapid rise in academic journals implementing this policy and the removal of editors who object.

'The publisher Elsevier has produced a template of author instructions for their 2,900 journals using the phrase "sex assigned at birth" and stating sex is not binary. Authors are also required to complete a survey during manuscript submission that presumes gender identity is a universal characteristic and includes no option to indicate the concept does not apply. Thus, Elsevier institutionalises not just desexed language but forces the concept of gender identity on all authors, irrespective of location, culture, or beliefs.'

'Relatedly, some ethics committees are discouraging researchers from collecting data on sex, adversely affecting efforts toward closing the female data gap. In some cases, such guidance was developed by diversity and inclusion sections of universities.'[9]

A study published in 2024, including thousands of people and 15 states in America, concluded that American anti-transgender legislation increased the possibility of suicide; but, it turns out, the main evidence did not come from the study as a whole, but a questionable sub-group in Idaho. What is more, 'This raises an obvious question: if the policies cited as the source of harm were never fully operational, can they plausibly be identified as the cause of the reported outcomes?'[10]

Therefore, the question of whether or not WPATH citations are valid, is anything but settled fact. Indeed, if this account of the policy of editors, journals, and ethics committee's is as widespread as has been reported in Gribble's article, then it is clear that WPATH's referring to sixty-nine pages of citations does not answer the question of whether or not this is supporting evidence or a smoke screen, deterring all but the most determined and well informed to question it.

---

[9] Karleen Gribble, 3rd March, 2026, "Erasing the Word "Woman": The desexing of language in women's health research and care is a story of the marginalisation of science, cultural imperialism, and abuse of power: https://quillette.com/2026/03/03/erasing-the-word-woman-trans-healthcare-mothers-breastfeeding/.

[10] August 12th, 2026, "Do Laws Restricting Gender Transition Increase Youth Suicide? A New Scientific Challenge to a Widely Repeated Narrative": https://zenit.org/2026/08/12/do-laws-restricting-gender-transition-increase-youth-suicide-a-new-scientific-challenge-to-a-widely-repeated-narrative/?eti=34714.

However, destroying a healthy sexual organ, such as a vagina, by turning it into a facsimile of a male sexual organ, does not require pages of 'guidance' to see that it is a harmful practice; and, therefore, whatever these 'scientific studies' claim, the bare fact is that a person's bodily, sexual organ, whether that person is young or old, has been mutilated: it has been rendered unfit for use, in terms of its original shape and function, and cannot be restored to that original shape and function. Similarly, for what happens to a male organ turned into a facsimile of a female opening. In other words, these surgical processes are expensive, irreversible wounds.

### *The Questioning of Decision Making*

The question of whether or not a doctor has been 'duped'[11] can be answered concretely by a doctor who carried out the removal of healthy wombs and then began to question on what authoritative basis she was doing it. And, it seems, what was a part of this doctor questioning what she was doing was the sense that there was a process by which "medical permission" was given for this procedure but that, on examination, this doctor found that there was no medical basis for this procedure at all.[12] The claim that distress about a person's sexuality warrants a radically body-altering and mutilating procedure is simply that, a claim; but, it is not just a claim, it is a course

---

[11] Case No. 4:26-cv-00748-O. DEFENDANT WORLD PROFESSIONAL ASSOCIATION FOR TRANSGENDER HEALTH, INC.'S MEMORANDUM IN SUPPORT OF ITS MOTION TO DISMIS, pp. 1 and8-9.

[12] Dr. Karla Solheim, MD, FACOG, May 27th, 2025, "It's Time for Liberal Physicians to Rethink American Gender Medicine: The Ethics of the Gender Affirming Hysterectomy".

of action that renders a girl or young woman sterile. And, indeed, there are many other experts who, as professionals, object to the transition from health to infertility[13].

In the previous book, book two of this series, I discussed extensively the mentality of "letting the child decide", as if there is no clinical responsibility on the part of the clinicians, advisers, and the people in the program who progressively authorize actions from a change of name to surgery. But, as we can see, there is a whole train of professionals involved in a decision-making process which, it can be argued, unethically claims that a child can make a life-altering decision about his or her body parts. This abdication of professional responsibility, at every step, is part of the problem, not the solution.

Who is responsible for the use of an endocrine prescription which allows the prescribing of doses of hormones beyond the scale of even what a genuinely medical treatment requires?

### *Marketing or Guidance?*

Thirdly, the 'Defendant[,] the World Professional Association for Transgender Health ("WPATH") does not make statements to consumers at all.'[14] Are not doctors and the general public 'consumers' in this context as they act on the basis of a presumed authoritative judgement in cases of gender dysphoria? What is more, the general

---

[13] *Cf. Transgenderism Two: Evidence and Identity*: https://enroutebooksandmedia.com/transgenderismtwo/.

[14] Case No. 4:26-cv-00748-O. DEFENDANT WORLD PROFESSIONAL ASSOCIATION FOR TRANSGENDER HEALTH, INC.'S MEMORANDUM IN SUPPORT OF ITS MOTION TO DISMIS, p. 1.

work of transgender assessment, medicalization, and surgical intervention, are all paid activities. Indeed, claiming insurance cover for these medical interventions indicates that these are "commercial transactions" and not merely "medical guidance" with no pecuniary consequence. However, what is very striking is that WPATH consistently "distances" itself from any action that implements gender ideology that can be attributed to its "SOC-8" guidance. At the same time, "SOC-8" guidance seems to target what is characterized as 'conversion therapy'[15] which, historically, was an objectionable practice. But American law defends the right to free speech and thus 'the Court struck down a law prohibiting a therapist from providing talk-based conversion therapy.'[16] The question arises, however, as to why 'providing talk-based conversion therapy' is of itself objectionable unless, that is, it is construed *a priori* as a type of verbal or physical violence; and, if it is construed *a priori* then it is not because of an actual discernment as that it is a historical stereotype being used, manipulatively, in the present, to object to legitimate talk therapy. However, when it comes to verbal violence, is not the claim, "Do you want a live daughter or a dead son?", a type of reprehensible 'conversion therapy'? Indeed, does WPATH reject the gender ideologist's

[15] E. Coleman, A. E. Radix, W. P. Bouman, et al. (2022) Standards of Care for the Health of Transgender and Gender Diverse People, Version 8, International Journal of Transgender Health, 23:sup1, S1-S259, DOI, cites a negative view of 'conversion therapy' 24 times and, as such, does not distinguish between an exploratory type therapy which could result in a person being reconciled to their original sex and a type of reprehensible talk therapy that is genuinely a kind of verbal violence.

[16] Case No. 4:26-cv-00748-O. DEFENDANT WORLD PROFESSIONAL ASSOCIATION FOR TRANSGENDER HEALTH, INC.'S MEMORANDUM IN SUPPORT OF ITS MOTION TO DISMIS, p. 34.

type of 'conversion therapy' that is used in the name of 'gender-affirming care' to affirm whatever a child calls him or herself?

What is of note, too, is that there have been relatively longstanding medical codes for those who wanted to 'transition', so there is available money to pay for it; and, in addition, it is only because of these insurance claims that it has been possible to trace some of the people who went through these procedures. Why, if WPATH is concerned with evidence-based medicine, has there not been proper record-keeping of the people, especially young people, who have been through gender clinics, so that there can be a proper assessment of how many have gone through, what the long-term outcomes are, and how many have regretted it?[17] Or is it claimed that there is no connection between WPATH and what happens in gender clinics? But isn't this part of patient feedback that informs patient care? Notably, then, it is only now that there are American codes, published by the American Centre for Disease Control (CDC) for the 'detransitioner' which, hopefully, will start to give a factual basis to this under recorded phenomenon; these codes, then can entail detailing medical histories, and will mean that 'physicians will be able to more accurately document an individual's clinical state to support the appropriate delivery of care.'[18]. If, again, gender ideologists are advocating evidence-based care, why has there been resistance to introducing codes that can show how many people regret what has happened

[17] The Cass Report was particularly critical of the UK National Health Service's lack of records.

[18] "Do No Harm", August 13th, 2026, "Why the CDC's New ICD-10 Codes Matter for Detransitioners": https://donoharmmedicine.org/2026/08/13/ why-the-cdcs-new-icd-10-codes-matter-for-detransitioners/.

to them: 'Right now, nobody knows how many people want to reclaim their true gender, because the system was originally designed to ignore them.'[19]

'The Fifth Circuit has held that "merely publishing a medical opinion—even a hotly debated one— in a peer-reviewed journal cannot give rise to a misrepresentation claim."[20] But publishing 'guidance' is different to publishing so called 'peer-reviewed' articles? What is more, the claim at issue is that this guidance was authoritative on the basis that this organization's claim is to be *the authoritative* voice in this so-called area of medicine. In terms of guidance, then, has WPATH distanced itself from the following practices? Do you want a dead son or daughter or a live daughter or son? Are they encouraging young people to use special words and to espouse views that were clearly not their own but an expression of an ideological take on certain fluctuating reactions in the course of growing up? In other words, the whole language used in parental-child dialogues was manipulative and aimed at the goal of persuading a child to "transition" and a parent to agree to it.

---

[19] AIDA CERUNDOLO, MD, 08/13/26 7:30 AM ET, « CDC HAS MADE SURE DETRANSITIONERS ARE NO LONGER INVISIBLE": HTTPS://THEHILL.COM/OPINION/HEALTHCARE/5992273-CDC-ADDS-DETRANSITIONER-CODES/.

[20] Case No. 4:26-cv-00748-O. DEFENDANT WORLD PROFESSIONAL ASSOCIATION FOR TRANSGENDER HEALTH, INC.'S MEMORANDUM IN SUPPORT OF ITS MOTION TO DISMIS, p. 1.

### *Conclusion: Soft Changes with Hard Outcomes*

Clearly the "SOC-8" document, and other WPATH documents, are very carefully worded. However, even in its discussion on prepubertal children, in "SOC-8", which it recognizes will not necessarily continue on a transgender trajectory, the authors draw back from linking being transgender with the overwhelming cultural influences which now exist in our society. In other words, while the authors repeatedly refer to transphobia and other negative influences[21], they seem "immune" to recognizing that the growth in "transgenderism" is itself a cultural phenomenon which correlates with the rise of social media, exposure to these kinds of ideas in chats with those who endorse them, and that being transgender is not, therefore, some kind of "new" discovery but, rather, one that is a function of advocacy over many years.

It is therefore too simplistic to claim that ""[P]repubescent gender diverse children," however, "are not eligible to access medical intervention" at all. SOC-8 at S67.'[22] More widely, if the program of change begins with pronouns and other, "soft changes", it is not so much about whether 'medical intervention' is available then as that the gender-affirming-care program moves towards it. More widely, then, it is essential to establish the truth of what is happening in the

---

[21] Cf. E. Coleman, A. E. Radix, W. P. Bouman, et al. (2022) Standards of Care for the Health of Transgender and Gender Diverse People, Version 8, International Journal of Transgender Health, 23:sup1, S1-S259, DOI: 10.1080/26895269.2022.2100644: Chapter 7.

[22]Case No. 4:26-cv-00748-O. DEFENDANT WORLD PROFESSIONAL ASSOCIATION FOR TRANSGENDER HEALTH, INC.'S MEMORANDUM IN SUPPORT OF ITS MOTION TO DISMIS, pp. 5-6.

course of 'gender-affirming-care' so that medical treatment is not based on ideologically actioned, political activism[23].

### *A Lasting word*

The final word, however, goes to God and to Holy Scripture: that even if we do not know when to stop, there is a stopping point appointed by God, namely the help advocated by the Son of God to bring forgiveness and mercy to all: 'Jesus said, "Father, forgive them; they do not know what they are doing"' (Luke 23: 34). Let us note, too, that human beings often do not know that what they want is beyond their power to action; and, therefore, we need to listen to the wisdom of the word of God which says: 'the nations shall know that that they are no more than human' (Psalm 9: 20). Let us remember, too, that sometimes we want what is not possible, whereas other things are only possible with divine help. Let us pray, therefore, for that discernment that may lead us to find a way forward that both protects our young people and recognizes that sex is not an invention but a gift: that the existence of male and female (cf. Genesis 1: 27) is both an expression of a religious truth and a naturally evident, empirical fact: that the complementary difference between male and female is foundational for many, if not all species. Thus, let all, on

---

[23] Cf. "Wolves in White Coates: How Doctors and Hospitals Pushed and Profited from the Fraud of "Gender Medicine"", 2026, Make America Healthy Again: https://www.hhs.gov/sites/default/files/hhs-wolves-in-white-coats.pdf. Pp. 1-27: Note the sheer political advocacy of gender ideology under the Biden Administration; and, therefore, the question arises: Why did the Biden Administration do this? Were there outside money incentives to do this? Were there pressure groups advocating this?

whatever stage of the journey we are on[24], not remain isolated, sidelined, or lost – but continue on in the search for the truth, lovingly expressed.

[24] The history of Israel is replete with journeys, particularly in the life of Abraham and in the Exodus from Egypt but in many other times and places too, including the New Testament.

## Prayer to the Holy Family for help

Dear God and Father of mankind,
help us to investigate all that you have done,
both throughout the natural world and, more especially,
through the breadth and depth of the human person,
male or female –
but let us be open, too, to the work
of a word-grace given to help us.

Dear Lord, Jesus Christ,
you came in the flesh of our humanity,
born through the faith of your Holy Mother,
the Virgin Mary, born to transfigure our wounded nature,
healing and opening it upon the horizon of heaven that we,
often imperfect, scarred, bitter, and sinful,
may begin to rejoice in the gift of life,
given to us and given to all, that
we might be born into an ever-fuller life here
and to eternal life in the hereafter.

Dear Holy Spirit, how many and how diverse
are the paths from evidence to truth,
from reason to further reflection,
from Revelation to understanding the mystery of mysteries
as we contemplate our selves in the mirror of the Blessed Trinity:

Send us a new spirit of enquiry,
a new openness to the discoverable truth,
a new willingness to persevere when our way is
blocked, derailed, hopeless, painful and even
nearing a dead end, so that we may see anew
that coming to the point of endless disappointments is
the place of your help:

My Mary, Our Mother, Joseph, and the Lord Jesus,
Intercede for the family in this generation.

Amen.

www.ingramcontent.com/pod-product-compliance
Lightning Source LLC
LaVergne TN
LVHW021737071126
851857LV00040B/1474